INDIAN SPICES & CONDIMENTS AS

NATURAL HEALERS

INDIAN SPICES & CONDIMENTS AS

NATURAL HEALERS

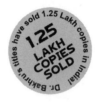

DR. H. K. BAKHRU

NATIONALLY ACCLAIMED NATUROPATH

JAICO PUBLISHING HOUSE

Ahmedabad Bangalore Bhopal Bhubaneswar Chennai
Delhi Hyderabad Kolkata Lucknow Mumbai

Published by Jaico Publishing House
A-2 Jash Chambers, 7-A Sir Phirozshah Mehta Road
Fort, Mumbai - 400 001
jaicopub@jaicobooks.com
www.jaicobooks.com

INDIAN SPICES & CONDIMENTS
AS NATURAL HEALERS
ISBN 81-7224-831-8

First Jaico Impression: 2001
Seventh Jaico Impression (Reformatted): 2011

Printed by
Kaveri Printers Pvt. Ltd.
19, Ansari Road, Darya Ganj
New Delhi - 110 002

About the Author

Dr. H.K. Bakhru enjoys a countrywide reputation as an expert naturopath and a prolific writer. His well-researched articles on nature cure, health, nutrition and herbs appear regularly in various newspapers and magazines and they bear the stamp of authority.

A diploma holder in naturopathy, all his current 13 books on nature cure, nutrition and herbs titled, *A Complete Handbook of Nature Cure, Diet Cure for Common Ailments, A Handbook of Natural Beauty, Nature Cure for Children, Naturopathy for Longevity, Healing Through Natural Foods, Indian Spices and Condiments as Natural Healers, Foods That Heal, Herbs That Heal, Natural Home Remedies for Common Ailments, Vitamins that Heal, Conquering Diabetes Naturally* and *Conquering Cancer Naturally* have been highly appreciated by the public and repeatedly reprinted. His first-named book has been awarded first prize in the category *'Primer on Naturopathy for Healthy Living'* by the jury of judges at the *'Book Prize Award'* scheme, organized by *National Institute of Naturopathy*, an autonomous body under Govt. of India, Ministry of Health.

Dr. Bakhru began his career on the Indian Railways, with a first class first postgraduate degree in History from Lucknow

University in 1949. He retired in October 1984 as the Chief Public Relations Officer of the Central Railway in Mumbai, having to his credit 35 years of distinguished service in the Public Relations organisations of the Indian Railways and the Railway Board.

An associate member of the All India Alternative Medical Practitioner's Association and a member of the Nature Cure Practitioners' Guild in Mumbai, Dr. Bakhru has extensively studied herbs and natural methods of treating diseases. He has been honoured with 'Lifetime Achievement Award', 'Gem of Alternative Medicines' award and a gold medal in Diet Therapy by the Indian Board of Alternative Medicines, Calcutta, in recognition of his dedication and outstanding contributions in the field of Alternative Medicines. The Board, which is affiliated with the Open International University for Complementary Medicines, established under World Health Organisation and recognised by the United Nations Peace University, has also appointed him as its Honorary Advisor. Dr. Bakhru has also been honoured by Nature Cure Practitioners' Guild, Mumbai with Nature Cure Appreciation Award for his services to Naturopathy.

Dr. Bakhru has founded a registered Public Charitable Trust, known as D.H. Bakhru Foundation, for help to the poor and needy. He has been donating Rs. 25,000 every year to this trust from his income as writer and author.

Dr. Bakhru spends his retired life, devoting all his time to the furtherance of the cause of nature cure and charitable activities under the auspices of the Trust.

Contents

Preface

The history of Indian spices and condiments is probably as old as human civilisation itself. There are numerous references about them in the Vedas, the Bible and the Quran. The earliest literary record in India on spices and condiments is in the Rig Veda, around 6000 BC.

Indian spices have been famous since pre-historic times. Indian ships were carrying Indian spices and other products to Mesopotamia, Arabia and Egypt, centuries before Greece and Rome had their birth. This attracted many seafarers to come to the shores of India.

The Greek merchants thronged the markets of South India to purchase the spices, besides other precious articles like diamonds and textiles, long before the Christian era. Romans, who were fond of sensuous pleasures, were spending huge amounts on Indian spices and other famed Indian products. It is said that there might have been no crusades and no expeditions to the East without the lure of Indian spices and other famed products.

In spite of the industrial advancement of India in modern times, this country is still regarded as the Home Of Spices.

This is due to the fact that the quality of the spices produced in and exported from this country continues to be one of the best. The international trade in spices has grown by leaps and bounds. An estimated 500,000 tonnes of spices and herbs valued at 1500 million US dollars are now imported globally every year. An impressive 46% of this supply comes from India. India's exports of spice extracts have shown spectacular growth, attaining over 50 per cent of the global market within a short span.

Spices and condiments are one of the most important forms of natural foods. Besides culinary uses, they have been used in indigenous systems of medicine as natural healers since ancient times. They thus form part of our heritage healing. This book describes in great detail the medicinal virtues of different spices and condiments, and their usefulness in the treatment of various common ailments. This information can serve as a guide to the readers to solve their common health problems through the use of specific spices and condiments, besides adopting a well-balanced natural diet. It would, however, be advisable to consult a doctor or an expert naturopath in case of serious illnesses.

Diseases that Respond to Sepcific Spices and Condiments

Spices/ Condiments	Diseases/ Conditions
1 Aniseed	Asthma, Cataract, Flatulence, Gas-formation, Head lice, Insomnia.
2 Asafoetida	Amnesia, Asthma, Bronchitis, Excessive and painful menstruation, Female sterility, Flatulence, Hysteria, Leucorrhoea, Premature labour, Sexual impotence, toothache, unwanted abortion, whooping cough.
3 Basil	Asthma, bad breath, Bronchitis, Cold, Constipation, Cough, Dysentery, Earache, Fever, Gout, Headache, Heart disease, High blood cholesterol, Influenza, Insect bite, leucoderma, mouth infection, Neuralgia, Piles, Pyorrhoea, Ringworm, Sinusitis, sore eyes, sore throat, stress.

		Asthma, Bronchitis, Cholera, Colic, Cold, Diarrhoea, Dysentery, Dyspepsia, Earache, Flatulence, Hoarseness, Influenza, Migraine
4	Bishop's Weed	Neuralgic pain, Pharyngitis, Sexual impotence, Throat congestion.
5	Caraway Seeds	Bad breath, Colic, Flatulence, Hookworms, Scabies.
6	Cardamom	Bad breath, Burning micturition, Cystitis, Depression, Gonorrhoea, Hiccups, Hoarseness, Indigestion, Nephritis, Pharyngitis, Scanty urination, Sexual impotence, Sore throat.
7	Celery Seeds	Asthma, Indigestion, Insomnia, Liver disorders, Rheumatism.
8	Chillies or Capsicums	Asthma, Blood clot, Bronchitis, Depression, Dyspepsia, Lumbago, Neuralgia, Pharyngitis, Rheumatic affliction, Sinusitis, Sore throat.
9	Cinnamon	Acne, Asthma, Bad breath, Cold, Diabetes, Diarrhoea, Excessive menstruation, Flatulence, Headache, Indigestion, Nausea, Paralysis, Sore throat, Vomiting.

10	Clove	Arthritis, Asthma, Blood clot, Bronchitis, Cholera, Colic, Earache, Food poisoning, Headache, Indigestion, Migraine, Muscular cramp, Neuralgia, Pharyngitis, Sexual debility, Stye, Toothache, Tuberculosis.
11	Coriander	Acidity, Acne, Colitis, Conjunctivitis, Dry skin, Dysentery, Excessive Menstruation, Fever, Hepatitis, High blood cholesterol, Indigestion, Small pox.
12	Cumin Seeds	Amnesia, Biliousness, Boils, Cold, Colic, Diarrhoea, Dyspepsia, Flatulence, Insomnia, Morning sickness, Piles, Scorpion sting.
13	Curry Leaves	Burns and bruises, Diabetes, Diarrhoea, Dysentery, Insect bite, Morning sickness, Nausea, Premature greying of hair, Vomiting.
14	Dill	Acidity, Bad breath, Boils, Bronchitis, Cold, Colic, Constipation, Diarrhoea, Dysentery, Hiccup, Influenza, Insomnia, Painful Menstruation.
		Asthma, Biliousness, Bronchitis, Colic, Conjunctivitis, Constipation,

15 Fennel	Cough, Dyspepsia, Flatulence, Menstrual irregularities, Painful menstruation, Vomiting.
16 Fenugreek	Anaemia, Bad breath, Biliousness, Body odour, Bronchitis, Colic, Dandruff, Diabetes, Diarrhoea, Dry skin, Dysentery, Dyspepsia, Fever, Flatulence, High blood cholesterol, Influenza, Leucorrhoea, Mouth ulcers, Pneumonia, Premature wrinkles, Sinusitis, Sore throat, Swelling.
17 Garlic	Arthritis, Asthma, Blood clot, Blood disorders, Boils, Cancer, Cholera, Cold, Cough, Depression, Diabetes, Diarrhoea, Diphtheria, Dysentery, Earache, Encephalitis, Genital herpes, Heart disease, Herpes virus, High blood cholesterol, High blood pressure, Influenza, Lumbago, Middle-ear infection, Peptic ulcer, Pneumonia, Ringworm, Sexual impotence, Tuberculosis, Typhoid, Verrucae, Whooping cough, Wounds.
	Arthritis, Asthma, Blood clot, Bronchitis, Chest congestion, Cholera, Cold, Colic, Cough, Diarrhoea, Dyspepsia, Earache, Flatulence, Headache, Influenza, Migraine, Nausea, Painful

18 Ginger	menstruation, Rheumatic affliction, Sexual impotence, Toothache, Tuberculosis, Vomiting, Whooping cough.
19 Liquorice	Alopecia (Patchy baldness), Cancer, Constipation, Corns, Cough, Muscular pains, Myopia, Oral inflammation, Peptic ulcer, Scalds, Sore throat, Stomach distress, Wounds.
20 Long Pepper	Asthma, Bronchitis, Cholera, Cold, Colic, Convulsions, Cough, Dyspepsia, Epilepsy, Gout, Hysteria, Insomnia, Menstrual irregularities, Muscular Pain, Rheumatism.
21 Marjoram	Asthma, Bruises, Cold, Colic, Diarrhoea, Flatulence, Scanty menstruation, Sprains, Stiff, Toothache.
22 Mint	Abdominal pain, Asthma, Biliousness, Bronchitis, Colic, Diarrhoea, Hoarseness, Indigestion, Morning sickness, Pyorrhoea, Thread worms, Tooth decay.
	Acne, Asthma, Bronchitis, Convulsion in children, Falling of

23	Mustard	hair, Muscular pains, Ringworm, Vomiting.
24	Nutmeg	Cold, Dehydration, Depression, Diarrhoea, Eczema, Hiccups, Indigestion, Insomnia, Morning sickness, Neuralgia, Ringworm, Rheumatic pain, Sciatica, Sexual impotence.
25	Onion	Anaemia, Arthritis, Blood clot, Bronchitis, Burning micturition, Cholera, Cold, Cough, Diabetes, Earache, Heart disease, High blood cholesterol, Influenza, Piles, Sexual impotence, Toothache, Tuberculosis, Urine retention, Warts.
26	Pepper	Amnesia, Cold, Cough, Dental caries, Digestive disorders, Muscular pains, Pyorrhoea, Sexual impotence, Toothache.
27	Poppy Seeds	Aches and Pains, Dysentery, Fevers, Insomnia, Itching.
28	Saffron	Bruises and Sores, Colic, Diabetes, Enlargement of liver and spleen, fevers, Hysteria, Leucorrhoea, Menstrual irregularities, Scanty urination.

29	Tamarind	Burns, Cold, Dysentery, Fevers, Flatulence, Indigestion, Inflammation of joints and ankles, Scurvy, Sore throat, Swellings, Vomiting.
30	Turmeric	Anaemia, Arthritis, Asthma, Boils, Cold, Cough, Diarrhoea, Flatulence, Influenza, Measles, Rhinitis, Ringworm, Scabies, Sore eyes, Sprains, Throat infection, Worms.

1

Aniseed

An Ideal Remedy for Flatulence

Description

Aniseed *(pimpinella anisum),* one of the oldest spices, is an annual plant, which grows to a height of 50 cms. It bears white flowers in summer. The fruits are small. The seeds are ground-grey to greyish-brown in colour, oval in shape and 3.2 to 4.8 mm in length. Five longitudinal ridges are visible on each pericarp. They have an agreeable odour and a pleasant taste.

Aniseed has often been mistaken for fennel, as common Indian name sauf applies to both. In European countries also, aniseed is sometimes mistaken with another spice 'star anise' which is, botanically different and is known as *Illicium verum.*

Star anise is indigenous to Southern China and TongKing and is extensively cultivated in those parts.

Origin and distribution

Anise is a native of the East Mediterranean region. The ancient Egyptians, who valued its medicinal properties and culinary uses, cultivated it. It was also known to the early

Greeks and Romans. It is now widely cultivated in Central and Southern Europe and all other tropical countries.

Anise is believed to have been introduced in India by the Mohammedan invaders from Persia. It is now grown in various parts of Uttar Pradesh and Punjab and, to a smaller extent, in Orissa. Though not a true native of the Indian soil, it is completely naturalised in the country at present.

Nutritive value/Composition

The origin of the aniseed determines its chemical composition. The ranges of values are: moisture 9-13 percent, protein 18 percent, fatty oil 8-23 percent, essential oil 2-7 percent, sugar 3.5 percent, starch 5 percent, crude fibre 12-25 percent and ash 6-10 percent. It also contains Choline.

Aniseed yields 2 to 3.5 percent of an essential oil which resembles Star-Anise. This oil is a colorless or pale-yellow liquid, with the characteristic odour and taste of the fruit. This oil has now replaced the fruits for medicinal and flavoring purposes.

The chief constituent of aniseed oil. is anethole, which is present to the extent of 80-90 percent, and is mainly responsible for the characteristic flavour of the oil and its sweet aromatic taste. The oil also contains methyl, chavicol, p-methoxyphenyl acetone and small amounts of terpenes and sulphur compounds of disagreeable odour. The anise spice cultivated in India yield the same constituents on distillation as the other varieties and are in no way inferior. Both the Anise oil and Star anise oil have been made official and can therefore, be used freely in medicine.

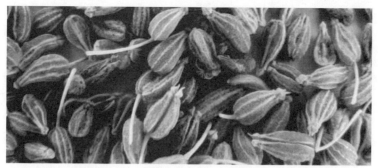

Aniseed relieves flatulence and removes catarrhal matter from the bronchial tubes.

Medicinal Virtues

Aniseed is favoured in medicine for it's properties to relieve flatulence and to remove catarrhal matter and phlegm from the bronchial tube. These properties are due to the presence of its essential oil. The seed also induces copious perspiration and increases the secretion and discharge of urine. The distilled water of anise is sold in Indian bazaars as 'araq badiari or 'araq sauf'. This water also possesses many medicinal virtues. The leaves of the plant are useful in relieving gas. They strenghthen the stomach and promote its action. They also possess mucus-clearing property.

• Flatulence

Aniseed possesses gas-relieving property. It is an excellent remedy for flatulence and it helps expel wind from the stomach. It can also be taken, in combination with other digestive foods like ginger, cumin and pepper, in the form of an infusion. Boiled with milk and a large cardamom, it is an excellent carminative for bottle-fed infants.

An easy way to prepare the infusion is to mix a teaspoon of aniseed in a cup of boiling water and leave it covered overnight. The clear fluid is then decanted and taken with honey. This helps relieve gurgling in the abdomen. It is also useful in preventing gas and fermentation in the stomach and the bowels.

Aniseed can also be taken in the form of tea for relieving flatulence. This tea is prepared as follows: Put about 325 ml. of water in a saucepan and bring to a boil. Add 1 teaspoon of aniseed, cover with a lid, lower the heat and simmer for 15 minutes. Strain and drink hot or warm. This tea can be sweetened with honey and hot milk can also be added to it. If ground aniseed is to be used, half the quantity of seeds should be used and the quantity of water should also be reduced by one-quarter.

A tea prepared from aniseed, caraway seed and fennel seed has also been found beneficial in the treatment of flatulence. This tea is prepared in the same manner as aniseed tea, using 500 ml. of water and 1 teaspoon each of the three seeds. A cupful of this tea should be sipped three times a day after meals. The left over tea should be kept covered in a cool place. The quantity required each time should be heated before use. If ground seeds are to be used, the quantity of the seeds should be reduced by one-quarter.

• Respiratory diseases

This spice is a valuable mucus-clearing food. It possesses expectorant property and helps remove phlegm from the bronchial tube. It contains the chemicals creosol and alpha-pinene, which is known to loose mucus in the bronchial tubes and make it easier to cough up. It can thus be beneficially used in respiratory system diseases like asthma, bronchitis and emphysema.

• Cataract

Aniseed is a useful remedy for cataract. Six grams of this spice should be taken daily in the morning and evening in treating this condition. As an alternative, aniseed and coriander seeds should be powdered together in equal quantities and mixed with an equal quantity of unrefined sugar. About 12 grams of this mixture should be taken in the morning and evening.

• Sleeplessness

Aniseed is a calming and sedative food. A tea made from this spice can calm the nerves and induce sleep. This tea can be prepared in the same manner as for relieving flatulence. It should be taken after meals or before going to bed.

• Women's problem

Traditional herbal healers have long recommended anise for secretion of breast milk in mother. Scientific studies have conformed this. Anise contains the compounds dianethole and photoanethole, which are chemically similar to the female hormone estrogen. In case of inadequacy of breast milk, nursing mothers should drink one cup of aniseed tea three times daily to increase breast milk. This tea also helps relieve menopausal symptoms like hot flashes. This is due to the same mild estrogenic action of aniseed that makes it valuable for nursing mothers.

Uses

Aniseed is mostly used as a flavouring agent to flavour curries, sweets, cakes, cookies and biscuits. Aniseed oil is employed in medicine as an aromatic carminative to relieve flatulence. Being a mild expectorant, it is used as an ingredient in beverages and liqueurs. It is a popular flavouring agent for dental preparations and mouth washes.

Precautions

Aniseed should not be boiled for a long time it may lose its digestive properties and essential oil during the process. Aniseed oil deteriorates on storage for a long period, especially if care is not taken to properly exclude light and air. It slowly loses its capacity to crystalline until, finally, it will no longer congeal. Anise oil should be used only when fresh. If it has solidified, it should be completely melted and mixed before use.

Asafoetida

A Sex Stimulant

2

Description

Asafoetida *(Ferula asafoetida)* is a dry latex or resinous gum of a tall perennial plant. This plant has massive taproot or carrot-shaped root, 12.5 to 15 cm in diameter at the crown, when they are 4 to 5 years old. The latex is collected in earthen vessels, dried and packed in leather bags in the form of hing. This process is usually done before the plant flowers. Asafoetida is murky yellow in colour, acrid and bitter in taste. It emits a strong, disagreeable, pungent, alliaceous odour due to the presence of sulphur compounds. Hence it is called 'Devil's dung' abroad. The odour of Asafoetida is stronger and more tenacious than that of the onion. It is used as a flavouring agent and forms a constituent of many spice mixtures.

Origin and distribution

Asafoetida has several varieties which are distributed from the Mediterranean region to Central Asia. It appears to have been introduced from East by the Arabian physicians. It is grown in Kandhar, Persia, Iran and Afghanistan. The other species, known botanically as Ferula narthex, grows abundantly in Kashmir, Western Tibet and Afghanistan. It forms a good substitute for asafoetida which is imported into India via the Khyber or Bolen passes or from the Persian Gulf ports. There are at least two types of asafoetida, one turning red and brownish on exposure to the air and the other type remaining pale buff or white.

Nutritive value/Composition

An analysis of asafoetida shows it to consist of moisture 16.0 percent, protein 4.0 percent, fat 1.1 percent, minerals 7.0 percent, fibre 4.1 percent and carbohydrates 67.8 percent per 100 grams. It's minerals and vitamin contents include calcium 690mg. percent, phosphorous 50 mg. percent, iron 39.4 mg. percent, carotene 4 mg. percent, riboflavin 0.04 mg. percent and niacin 0.3 mg. percent. Its calorific value is 297.

Asafoetida contains resin 40-64 percent, gum about 25 percent, volatile oil 10-17 percent and ash 1.5-10 percent. The resin consists chiefly of asaresinotennol, free or combined with ferulic acid. Umbelliferone seems to be present in the combined state. The oil of asafoetida is obtained by steam distillation of the gum resin. The yield of oil varies from 3 to 20 percent.

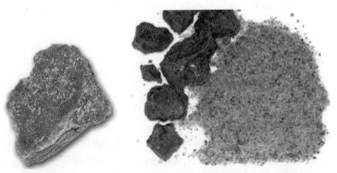

Asafoetida expels wind from the stomach and counteracts spasmodic disorders.

Medicinal virtues

Asafoetida has been widely used in indigenous system of medicines from the earliest times in India. It has been attributed properties to expel wind from the stomach and counteract many spasmodic disorders. It is also a nervine stimulant, digestive agent and a sedative. Recent studies have shown that asafoetida oil has antibiotic properties and inhibits growth of microbes.

In the body, asafoetida is absorbed from intestines and due to various volatile oils, it is excreted through lungs, skin and kidneys, leaving a sedative effect. It excites the secretion of ovarian hormones and sex stimulating centres.

• Digestive disorders

Asafoetida is a gas relieving food and an ideal medicine for several digestive disorders. It is one of the best medicines for expelling wind from the stomach. This spice has been found beneficial in the treatment of spasmodic disorders, indigestion and colic.

In case of flatulence and distension of the stomach, asafoetida should be dissolved in hot water and a pad of cloth soaked in it may be used for fomenting the abdomen. The spice can also be used beneficially as an enema for intestinal flatulence.

Adding asafoetida to foodstuffs, helps digestion and prevents flatulence by inhibiting the gas forming germs and eases the passage of flatus. Therefore, from ancient times in certain places of India, it is generally used along with every food, particularly with pickles and curries.

• Respiratory disorders

Asafoetida possesses expectorant property and it helps

remove catarrhs and phlegm from the bronchial tube. It thus helps control respiratory disorders like whooping cough, asthma and bronchitis. About 3 to 6 centigrams of this gum, should be taken mixed with 2 teaspoons of honey, a quarter teaspoon of white onion juice and 1 teaspoon of betel leaf juice, thrice daily. This mixture will be beneficial both for the prevention and treatment of these diseases. The smoke of asafoetida can be inhaled through a pipe to relieve the paroxysm of asthma.

• Infectious diseases

From ancient times, asafoetida is used as a preventive medicine for infectious diseases. In olden days, it used to be tied in a cloth and left hanging in one of the corners of the house. It was believed that the smell that emitted from the stuff was responsible for preventing the diseases. Perhaps the volatile oils and the smell might have influence on micro-organisms.

• Aches and pains

This spice possesses painkilling properties. Asafoetida 2 gms dissolved in one tablespoon of coconut oil, is applied as an analgesic balm in rheumatoid arthritis, mylagia and traumatic swelling. A paste of asafoetida, prepared with water or lime juice, is applied over wasp, bee, and scorpion stings. This spice is also a valuable remedy for relieving toothache. It should be pestled in lemon juice, and slightly heated. A cotton piece, soaked in the lotion should be placed in the cavity of the tooth. It will relieve pain quickly. The powder of the spice can also be applied with beneficial results on painful tooth and surrounding gums.

• Fevers (*Kala-Azar*)

The use of this spice has been found valuable in *Kala-Azar*, which is characterised by irregular fever, progressive anaemia and gradual increase in temperature. A small piece of asafoetida and one piece of garlic should be ground together. A drink made from this mixture should be taken once daily for a week in treating this disease. The same mixture should be applied as ointment over the spleen till it softens.

• Amnesia

This resinous gum is said to help regenerate the brain and the nervous system and thereby help increase memory. It also helps to tone up sluggish organs to create a feeling of youthful vitality. It can be used as a mind tonic in the powdered form. One and a half teaspoon of this powder should be dissolved in two cups of boiling water. It should be allowed to cool then sip several tablespoons while working. This gives a feeling of mental alertness and sharpens memory.

• Sexual impotence

Asafoetida is a powerful sex stimulating food. It is thus beneficial in the treatment of impotency. About 6 centigrams of this spice should be fried in ghee and mixed with honey and a teaspoon of fresh latex of banyan tree. This mixture should be taken once daily for 40 days before sunrise. It is also considered a specific medicine for spermatorrhoea and premature ejaculation.

• Hysteria

This spice is highly beneficial in the treatment of hysteria. In case of hysterial attacks, this resinous gum should be inhaled. When it is not possible to take oral doses, an emulsion made by 2 grams of the gum with 120 ml of water should be used as an enema per rectum.

• Intestinal worms

Asafoetida is also regarded in Ayurvedic, Chinese and Western medicine as an effective remedy for worms and other intestinal parasites. It can be administered as an enema for this purpose.

• Children's ailments

The use of asafoetida has been found valuable in the treatment of nervous disorders of children. In olden days in Europe, a small piece of this gum was hung around a child's neck, to protect it from any diseases, especially germs which are sensitive to its particular odour.

• Women's problems

Asafoetida is considered useful in the treatment of several problems concerning women such as sterility, habitual abortion, premature labour, unusually painful, difficult and excessive menstruation and leucorrhoea. About 12 centigrams of gum fried in ghee, mixed with 120 grams of goat's fresh milk and a tablespoon of honey, should be given thrice daily for a month. It excites the secretion of progestrone hormone.

For habitual abortion, six gms of asafoetida should be ground with water and 60 pills prepared. The woman with the tendency for habitual abortion should take one pill each twice a day, from the time of conception. The number of pills should be increased gradually till she takes 10 pills a day. The number should then be gradually reduced. This spice is also useful for woman after childbirth. Its use will keep her free from gas formation and other digestive problems owing to its antiflatulent and digestive properties. It is a normal practise in southern India to give the powder of this spice mixed with rice to woman after delivery. The use of asafoetida during this period also increases breast-milk. It should be given in doses of six centigrams with a teaspoon of infusion of cloves thrice daily for this purpose.

• Antidote of opium

This spice is used as an antidote of opium. Given in the same quantity as opium ingested by the patient, it will counteract the effect of the drug.

Uses

The gum resin is relished as a condiment in India and Iran where it is used to flavour curries, meatballs, dal and pickles. It is used in Europe and the United States in perfumes and for flavouring. The whole plant is used as a fresh vegetable.

Precaution

Asafoetida should not be used in excess, due to its semi-toxic effects. Infants and children in particular should not be given asafoetida in oral form, because it causes severe vomiting leading to dehydration.

Basil

A Remedy for Fevers

3

Description

The basil *(Ocimum basilicum)*, also known as sweet basil, is a well-known common plant of India. It is an erect, much-branched, smooth, stout, and aromatic plant 30-90 cm. high. It is an annual plant of the mint family. The plant bears clusters of small, white or pale purple, two-lipped flowers in raceme fashion.

The fresh leaves are bright green in colour and about 3.75 cm. in length. When dried, they turn brownish-green and brittle. Dried leaves and tender stems of this plant are used as a spice for flavouring and extraction of essential oils. The leaves have numerous dot-like oil glands which contains the aromatic oil of the herb.

Sweet basil has an aromatic clove-like scent which is, somewhat saline in taste. It has a slightly sweetish flavour, which increases while cooking. There is a widespread belief in India that, if basil is planted around homes and temples, it would ensure happiness.

There are numerous varieties of basil. Of these, four are identified in India. They are lettuce-leaf basil, curly-leafed basil, violet red basil and common white basil. Curly-leafed basil is considered most suitable for cultivation and it is reported to give good yields of high quality oil. It can be easily grown at home or in gardens in ordinary soil.

Origin and distribution

Basil is indigenous to the lower hills of Punjab and Himachal Pradesh and is cultivated throughout India. It was introduced into Europe in the sixteenth century and plants were established in english monastery gardens at about the same time. It is now cultivated in southern France and other Mediterranean countries and also in the USA. It grows abundantly in the warm climate of India, but sparingly in the cooler European weather.

Nutritive value/Composition

According to analysis report of the American Spice Trade Association (ASTA), USA, the composition of Basil is as follows:

moisture 6.1 percent, protein 11.9 percent, fat (Ether extract)3.6 percent, fibre 20.5 percent, carbohydrates 41.2 percent, total ash 16.7 percent, calcium 2.1 percent, phosphorous 0.47 percent, sodium 0.04 percent, potassium 3.7 percent and iron 0.04 percent. Its vitamin contents are thiamine 0.15 mg. percent, niacin 6.90 mg. percent, riboflavin 0.32 mg. percent, ascorbic acid 61.3 mg. percent and vitamin A 290 International units/ 100g. It contains 325 calories per 100g of dried herb.

A good commercial sample of sweet basil has been found to contain a minimum of 0.4 percent of volatile oil. This oil is produced by the distillation of the herb. The flowers, on an average, yield 0.4 percent oil while the whole plant contains 0.10 to 0.25 percent oil. The maximum total ash is 15 percent, maximum acid insoluble ash 1 percent, maximum moisture

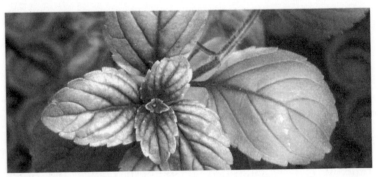

The leaves of basil are nerve tonic and they sharpen the memory

8 percent and total and minimum ether extract 4 percent on moisture-free basis.

Medicinal virtues

The powdered leaves of Basil were originally added to snuff to help clear the nostrils. The early herbalists also used this plant for soothing headaches and helping cure digestive ailments. Today it is used in digestive and nerve tonics, since it contains all the minerals and some Vitamin B.

The leaves and seeds of the plant possess curative properties. The leaves are nerve tonic and they sharpen the memory. They promote the removal of catarrhal matter and phlegm from the bronchial tubes. The leaves strengthen the stomach and promote its action and they also expel wind from the stomach. They induce copious perspiration. The seeds of the plant are mucilaginous and nourishing. They are stimulant and cooling. They exercise soothing effect on the skin and mucus membranes. They also increase the secretion and discharge of urine.

• Fevers

The leaves of basil are specific for many fevers. During the rainy season, when malaria and dengue fever are widely prevalent, a decoction of the tender leaves act as a preventive against these diseases. It should be given with ginger and white pepper in remittent and intermittent fevers. In case of acute fevers, the patient should be given a decoction of the leaves boiled with powdered cardamom in half a litre of water and mixed with honey or jaggery and milk. This brings down the temperature.

• Respiratory system disorders

The leaves are useful in respiratory system disorders. Their decoction, with honey and ginger is an effective remedy for bronchitis, asthma, influenza, cough arid cold. A decoction of the leaves, cloves and common salt also gives immediate relief in case of influenza. They should be boiled in half a litre of water till only half the water is left.

• Digestive system disorders

This spice helps counteract the effects of unwholesome food and is an aid to digestion. It is also a valuable remedy for nausea and vomiting. An infusion of the green leaves in boiling water can be used beneficially in treating these conditions.

• Genito-Urinary system disorders

The seeds of the plant can be used beneficially in the treatment of bladder infection and gonorrhoea. A teaspoon of the seeds mixed in a glass of water with some jaggery or honey makes an excellent medicine for treating these diseases.

• Constipation

The seeds of the plant act as a laxative. They can be taken

internally with beneficial results in case of habitual constipation and piles, which usually results from chronic constipation.

• Sinus trouble

The seeds of the plant have been found to be beneficial in the treatment of sinus problems. They can be used in the form of poultice for this purpose.

• As an insecticide

Basil oil possesses insecticidal and insect repellent properties. It is effective against house-flies and mosquitoes. It is also bactericidal.

• Women's problem

The mucilaginous jelly formed by infusing 1 to 3 drachms of the seeds in cold water for some time is given with jaggery or honey for relieving pains after childbirth.

• Stress

Basil leaves are regarded as adaptogen or anti-stress agent. Recent studies have shown that the leaves protect against stress significantly. It has been suggested that even healthy persons should chew 12 leaves of basil twice a day, morning and evening, for preventing stress. It will purify the blood and help prevent several common ailments.

• Skin diseases

The juice of basil leaf can be applied externally in case of ringworm and other skin diseases. It has also been tried successfully by some Naturopaths in the treatment of leucoderma.

• Tooth disorders

Basil leaves are beneficial in the treatment of tooth disorders.
They can be dried in the sun and powdered. This powder can
be used for brushing the teeth. It can also be mixed with
musturd oil to make a paste and used as tooth paste. It helps
maintain dental health and counteract foul smell. It is also
useful in pyorrhoea and other tooth disorders.

• Rheumatic afflictions

Basil is useful in rheumatic afflictions like gout joints. An
infusion of the plant can be given with beneficial results for
treating these conditions.

• Headache

Basil is useful in headache. A decoction of the leaves should
be given for treating this disorder. Pounded leaves mixed with
sandalwood paste can also be applied on the forehead for
getting relief from heat and headache. Dried basil leaves in
the form of snuff can also be used as a remedy for nervous
headaches and for relieving head colds.

• Earache

Basil leaves are also beneficial in the treatment of earache. A
few drops of the juice of the leaves should be put in the
affected ear to obtain relief. This remedy will also be useful
in the dullness of hearing.

• Body odour

The leaves of Basil have also been found beneficial in the
treatment of unpleasant body odour. About 20 leaves should
be eaten daily in the morning with a glass of water. This
treatment should be continued for a month or so.

• Croup

The use of this spice has been found valuable in croup, a disease marked by an obstruction in the larynx, mostly prevalent in children. The warm juice of the leaves should be taken in doses of half to one drachm, with honey in treating this condition. It has a slightly narcotic effect and allays irritation in the throat.

• Poisoning

The seeds of basil plant can be taken internally as an antidote to poison. They can also be applied externally on venomous bites.

Uses

Sweet basil is used as a flavouring agent in soups, fish, certain cheeses, tomato cocktail, eggplant, cooked cucumber dishes, cooked peas, squash and string beans. It is also used in the manufacture of chartreuse and other liquers. The oil of sweet basil is extensively used in all kinds of flavours, including confectionery, baked goods, condimentary products and in spiced meats and sausages. The oil also serves for imparting distinction to flavours in certain dental and oral products. Sweet basil oil is also used in certain perfume compounds and for the scenting of soaps.

4

Bishop's Weed
A Carminative Medicine

Description

Bishop's weed *(Trachyspermum ammi)* plant belongs to coriander family, and resembles dill plant. It is a small, erect, annual shrub which grows upto about 1 meter. It has soft fine hair. The stems of the plant are much branched and leafy. It has feather-like leaves 2.5 cm long; and 4 to 12 ray flowerheads, each bearing 6 to 16 flowers. The fruits are minute, egg-shaped and greyish.

The dry seeds are harvested in the form of *Ajwain seeds*. The seeds are egg-shaped about 2 mm. long and 1 mm. broad. There are five ridges over each seed with a depression in the middle. Inside the seed there are nine oil tubes that run vertically in them. The seeds are aromatic, sharp, tingling and slightly bitter. The colour of the seeds is greenish-brown.

Origin and distribution

The trade name *ajwain* is based on the Indian name, which is derived from *adarjawan*. Bishop's weed has been cultivated in India from ancient times. Besides India it is extensively cultivated in Iran, Egypt and Afghanistan. In India, it is largely grown in Uttar Pradesh, Bihar, Madhya

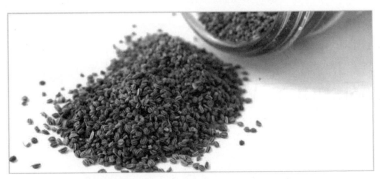

The seeds of Bishop's weed are stimulant and help counteract
spasmodic disorders

Pradesh, Punjab. Rajasthan, West Bengal, Tamil Nadu, and
Hyderabad.

Nutritive value/Composition

An analysis of the Bishop's weed shows it to consist of
moisture 7.4 percent, protein 17.1 percent, fat 21.8 percent,
minerals 7.9 percent, fibre 21.2 percent and carbohydrates
24.6 percent per 100 grams. The minerals and vitamins
contained in it are Calcium 1525 mg percent, phosphorus
443 mg percent, iron 12.5 mg percent, carotene 71 meg
percent, thiamin 0.21mg percent, riboflavin 0.28 mg percent
and niacin 2.1 mg percent. It's calorific value is 363.

The bishop's weed yields 2 to 3 percent of essential oil in
which thymol is present to the extent of 35 to 60 percent.
Thymol crystallises easily from the oil, and is sold in India as
ajwain-ka-phul (flowers of ajwain). The remainder of the oil
consists of pcymene, alpha-pinene, dipentine, alpha-terpentine,
and carvacrol. The oil of ajwain is almost colorless possesing
a characteristic odour and a sharp burning taste.

Medicinal virtues

Bishop's weed has been used as a carminative medicine from the time of Charaka and Sushruta, the great physicians of ancient India. The ancient Greek physicians like Dioscrides and Gelen also used it in various carminative medicines. Some very valuable Unani medicines are prepared from ajwain seeds.

The seeds are stimulant and are useful in counteracting spasmodic disorders. Ajwain oil, both pure and dethymolised, is used as an antiseptic and aromatic carminative in India. Its action and uses are similar to thymol which is a powerful antiseptic and finds varied application in medicine. The leaves of the plant are used as a vermicide. Even the roots of ajwain plant are reported to be diuretic and carminative.

• Digestive disorders

Bishop's weed has long been used in indigenous medicine for the treatment of various digestive disorders including flatulence and indigestion. For expelling gas from the stomach, the seeds may be eaten with betel leaves. A teaspoon of these seeds with a little rock salt is a household remedy for indigestion and gas formation. For indigestion, a tablespoon of seeds can also be boiled in a litre of water and this water drunk after adding a pinch of black salt. For stomachache, cough and indigestion, the seeds are masticated, swallowed and followed by a glass of hot water. For relieving colic pain a paste of the seeds should be locally applied to obtain relief.

A pinch of plain *ajwain* seeds one pinch are given along with jaggery as a folk medicine to prevent indigestion, and gastrointestinal infection after child birth.

The volatile oil extracted from the seeds is also useful in indigestion and gas formation. It is usually given in doses of

1 to 3 drops. *Ovam* water, the water distilled from the seeds, is an excellent carminative that can be used beneficially to relieve flatulence. It is antispasmodic in colic and flatulent dyspepsia.

Another effective remedy for flatulence is to soak bishop's weed and dried ginger in equal weight in two-and-half times the quantity of lime juice. This mixture should then be dried and powdered with a little black salt. About two grams of this powder should be taken with warm water in treating this condition.

• Respiratory disorders

This spice is a mucus clearing food and hence highly beneficial in the treatment of respiratory diseases. A mixture of the seeds and buttermilk is an effective remedy for relieving difficult expectoration caused by dried up phlegm. The seeds are also efficacious in bronchitis. A hot fomentation with the seeds is a popular household remedy for asthma.

A decoction of the *ajwain* seeds is an effective expectorant during the treatment of tuberculosis, asthma, bronchitis and lung abscess. This decoction is prepared by boiling a teaspoonful each of *ajwain* seeds and fenugreek seeds in a glass of water for half an hour. About 30 ml. of this decoction should be mixed with a tablespoonful of honey and taken thrice daily in treating this condition.

• Viral disease

Bishop's Weed is an anti-viral food. It is an effective remedy for cold. It has a remarkable power to open up clogged and congested nasal passages. A tablespoon of seeds crushed and tied up in a cloth can be used for inhalation. A similar bundle placed near the pillow, while sleeping, also relieves nasal congestion. For infants, a small pouch can be pinned to their dress under the chin when they are sleeping. In case of adults, a teaspoon of seeds can be put in boiling water and the vapours inhaled.

The use of Bishop's weed has also been found beneficial in the treatment of cough caused by acute pharyngitis in influenza. A pinch of seeds should be chewed with common salt and a clove as a medicine for this purpose.

• Cholera

The use of Bishop's weed has been found beneficial in the treatment of cholera. Ajwain seeds and Caraway seeds should be boiled together and little black salt and Mint added to it. The patient should be given this drink at regular intervals. The more the patient drinks, the better. This will help reduce the severity of the disease.

• Migraine

The seeds are useful in the treatment of migraine and delerium. They should either be smoked or sniffed frequently to obtain relief.

• Rheumatism

The oil extracted from the seeds is beneficial in the treatment of rheumatic and neuralgic pains. It should be applied on the affected parts.

• Mouth disorders

An infusion of the seeds mixed with common salt is an effective gargle in acute pharyngitis, sore and congested throat and hoarseness of the voice due to colds and shouting.

• Skin disorders

The use of *ajwain* seeds has been found valuable in skin

disorders like ringworm, syphilis, scabies, urticaria and psoriasis. The seeds should be taken mixed with jaggery in treating these disorders. The paste of the seeds prepared with half the quantity of turmeric powder can also be applied beneficially over scabies.

• Earache

Bishop's weed possesses pain-killing property. It is especially beneficial in treating earache. About half a teaspoon of the seeds is heated in 30 ml. of milk till the essence of the seeds permeate the milk. The milk is then filtered and used as ear drops. It decreases congestion and relieves pain.

In case of pain caused by boils in the ear, 3 gms each of *ajwain* seeds and garlic are boiled together in 40 gms of sesame oil till they turn red. The oil is then strained and cooled to body temperature, and used as ear drops.

• Sexual debility

Bishop's Weed is credited with aphrodisiac properties and hence beneficial in the treatment of sexual debility. The seeds of this plant, combined with kernel of tamarind seeds make a very effective sex tonic. Both these seeds in equal quantities should be fried in pure ghee, powdered and preserved in airtight containers. A teaspoon of this powder, mixed with a tablespoon of honey, should be taken daily with milk before retiring. It will increase virility and cure premature ejaculation. This remedy is far more effective than many costly medicines. Moreover, it enables the semen to impregnate the women by the production of spermatoza in it. The use of this remedy will also bless the person with a healthy child.

• Insect bites

The leaves are beneficial in the treatment of insect bites. A poultice of these leaves should be applied on the affected parts.

• Muscular pains

Bishop's weed is a valuable remedy for muscular pains. The seeds should be fried in coconut oil and should be massaged as a liniment in treating this condition.

• Prolapse of the Uterus

Bishop's weed is beneficial in the treatment of prolapse of the uterus. Some seeds should be tied in a cloth and soaked in water for 24 hours. The bundle should then be taken out and water allowed to drain. Some oil should be applied on the cloth and the bundle heated on fire. The uterus should be pushed in and a hot compress should be given with the bundle. This treatment should be repeated 3 to 5 times a day.

Uses

The greyish brown fruits or seeds are used as a spice, in flavouring numerous foods, as anti-oxidants, preservatives and in medicine. The aqueous solution of thymol is an excellent mouthwash and thymol is a constituent of many toothpastes.

Precaution

The seeds of bishop's weed should not be used in excess, as their excessive use can cause dryness of the fluids, damages the eyes and reduces the secretion of milk and semen.

Caraway Seeds

An Excellent Body Cleaner

5

Description

The caraway *(Carum carvi)* is a biennial, aromatic plant. It has usually a fleshy root, which tastes somewhat like carrots, and is yellowish on the outside and whitish on the inside. It has slender, branched stem that attains a height of 0.5 to 0.6 meters. The plant has finely cut, ferny leaves like the foliage of carrots. They are divided into very narrow segments. The flowers are small and white and they are used in many flower arrangements. The fruit, when ripe, splits into narrow, elongated carpels 4 to 6.5 mm long, curved, pointed at the ends and have four longitudinal ridges on the surface.

The seeds, which are actually one-half a piece of the fruits of the plant, are brown in colour and hard and sharp to touch. They are widely used as a spice for culinary purposes. They are available whole or ground. They have pleasant odour, aromatic flavour, somewhat sharp taste and leave a somewhat warm feeling in the mouth.

Origin and distribution

The caraway seed is indigenous to Europe, parts of Asia, India and North Africa. It's qualities were recognised by the ancient Egyptians, Greeks and Romans. Caraway is mentioned in Ebers papyrus of 1552 B.C., a manuscript by the Greek herbalist Dioscorides, and tiny seeds were found in a pile of 5,000 year-old debri left by primitive Mesolithic lake dwellers in Switzerland. It was used extensively by the ancient Greeks and Romans. It has been mentioned in the 12th century German medical book and a 14th century English cookbook.

The seeds were widely used in the Middle Ages. They have been used for centuries in breads, cakes, and with baked fruit, especially roasted apples. Because caraway was said to prevent lovers from straying, it was once an essential ingredient in love potions. The seeds of caraway were prescribed for bringing bloom to the cheeks of pale-faced young maidens. The plant was also reputed to have power against evil.

Caraway is now grown in north and central Europe, extending to the Caucasus, Persia, Tibet and Siberia. In India, the caraway grows wild in the north Himalayan region. The spice is cultivated as a winter crop on the plains and a summer crop in Kashmir, Kumaon, Garhawal and Chamba at altitudes of 2,740 to 3,660 metres.

Nutritive value/Composition

An analysis of caraway seeds shows it to contain moisture 4.5 percent, protein 7.6 percent, fat 8.8 percent, carbohydrates 50.2 percent, ash 3.7 percent, calcium 1.0 percent, phosphorous 0.11 percent, sodium 0.02 percent, potassium 1.9 percent, iron 0.09 percent, thiamine 3.38 percent, riboflavin 0.38 percent, niacin 8.1 percent, vitamin C 12.0 mg. percent and vitamin A 580 I.U. per 100 grams. Its calorific value is 465 per 100 gram.

A valuable oil, containing 45-65 percent of carvone, is obtained from caraway seeds. This oil is colourless or pale yellow with a strong odour and flavour of the fruit. The

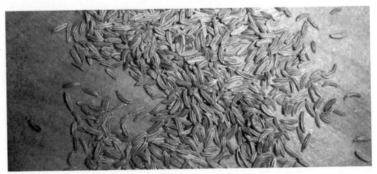

Caraway seeds form an excellent 'house cleaner' for the body.

volatile oil contains a mixture of ketone, carvone, terpene and traces of carvacrol.

Medicinal virtues

The caraway seeds, leaves and roots are considered useful in activating the glands, besides increasing the action of the kidneys. The seed is considered as an excellent 'house cleaner' for the body. The seeds, whole or ground help in the assimilation of starchy foods such as pastries, breads, biscuits, and certain vegetables which tend to produce flatulence such as cabbage, cucumber and onion. They also help digest stewed and baked fruits like apples and pears. Caraway oil is used in medicine to relieve flatulence. It is also used to correct the nauseating and gripping effects of some medicines.

• Digestive disorders

Caraway seeds are useful in strengthening the functions of stomach. They are gas relieving food and help expel wind from the stomach. They are useful in flatulent colic, and counter any possible adverse effects of medicines. However, the volatile oil of the seeds is employed more often than the seeds.

For flatulence, a cup of tea made from caraway seeds taken

thrice a day, after meals, will give relief. This tea is prepared by adding a teaspoon of caraway seeds in 1.5 to 2 litres of boiling water and allowing it to simmer on a slow fire for 15 minutes. It is then strained and sipped hot or warm.

• Hookworms

Carvone, isolated from caraway oil, is used as anthelmintic, especially in removing hookworms from the intestines.

• Scabies

A dilute solution, containing small amounts of the oil of the caraway and alcohol mixed in 75 parts of castor oil is considered beneficial in the treatment of scabies. The solution should be taken orally.

• Bad breath

Caraway seed oil is used orally in overcoming bad breath or insipid taste.

Uses

Today caraway is found in kitchens throughout the world. The roots and leaves can be used fresh. The long, slender roots are sometimes boiled as a vegetable and the leaves are sometimes used in salads, cream soups, cabbage, cauliflower potato dishes.

Caraway seeds, dried and whole are most often used as seasoning in rye bread. But a number of European countries like Germany, Holland, Austria, England and the Netherlands have long included it in their fare. Caraway seeds are widely used in biscuits and crackers, spiced seed cake, candies, cookies and cheese.

Cardamom

The Queen of Spices

6

Description

Cardamoms *(Elettaria cardamomum)* are broadly grouped into two categories, namely, small cardamom (Chhota elaichi) or true cardamom and large cardamom (Bara elaichi). The former is commercially far more important and also far more popular than the latter. In fact, it constitutes one of the most important and valued spices of the world. It is also the second most important 'national spice' of India, known as the 'Queen of Spices', being next to black pepper, called the 'King of Spices'. It is an indispensable part of everyday cooking.

Cardamom is a perennial plant with thick, fleshy branched rhizomes and several erect stems which sometimes grow upto a height of 3m. It has very large leaves, 30-90 cm. long, narrow with one strong median nerve and numerous faint side nerves.

The flowers are about 4 cm. long, white or pale green, borne in 30-90 cm. long bunches. The fruits are about 1.5 cm. long, pale green to yellow in colour, somewhat oval in shape, 3-celled and many-seeded.

The seeds are 2 to 3 mm. long angular in shape having pits

on them. Each seed is covered with a thin transparent colourless membrane, which becomes more prominent when moistened with water. The dried cardamom fruits of the plant contains medicinal virtues. They have a pleasant aroma and a characteristic warm and slightly pungent taste.

Origin and distribution

Cardamom is indigenous to Western Ghats in South India. It is mentioned by Theophrastus in the fourth century B.C. and later by Dioscorides in fifth century B.C. By 1000 A.D., it was an article of trade from India westwards.

Cardamom occurs wild in southern India, particularly in the moist forests of the hilly regions of Mysore and Kerala. It is also grown in adequate amounts in Sikkim. Cultivation of this spice is still limited to a few countries, mainly South India, Sri Lanka and Guatemala.

India exports about 90 percent of cardamom to the other exchange on this account. Indian cardamom is valued all over the world for its superior quality, unique flavour, rich content of oil, attractive shape and colour.

Nutritive value/Composition

Cardamom has excellent food value. It is low in fat and high in protein and vitamins A, B and C. An analysis of cardamom capsule shows it to consist of moisture 20 percent, protein 10.2 percent, ether extract 2.2 percent, volatile oil 7.4 percent, mineral matter (total ash) 5.4 percent, Crude fibre 20.1 percent, carbohydrates 42.1 percent, Calcium 0.13 percent, phosphorus 0.16 percent and iron 5 mg. percent per 100 grams. Its calorific value is 299.

The seeds contain 10 percent of volatile oil. The principal

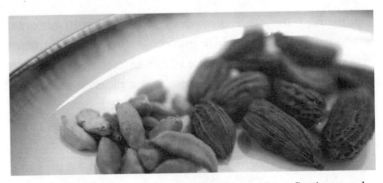

Cardamom are used chiefly in medicines to relieve flatulence and for strengthening digestion activities.

constituents of the oil are cineol, terpinene, limonene, sabinene and terpineol in the form of formic and acetic acid.

Medicinal virtues

The aroma and therapeutic properties of cardamom are due to its volatile oil. Tinctures of cardamom are also made. They are used chiefly in medicines for windiness and for strengthening the stomach. The medicinal virtues of cardamom were recognised even 2000 years ago. During the days of Charaka and Susrata the noted physicians of the 1st and 2nd centuries A.D., cardamom was acclaimed as a cure for many diseases. Today, the therapeutic value of this spice is widely recognised and Ayurvedic physicians use it for the treatment of various diseases. It is used as an adjunct to carminative drugs and is official in the British and U.S pharmacopoeias.

• Digestive disorders

Cardamom possesses carminative property. It helps subside the air and water elements in the body. It also increases appetite and soothes the mucus membranes. It relieves gas and heartburn and is useful in nausea and vomiting.

In case of gas formation in the stomach, half a teaspoon of this spice should be mixed in hot water and taken three times a day. Ground Cardamom seeds mixed with ginger, cloves and coriander are an effective remedy for indigestion. A decoction made from Cardamom has been found useful in headache resulting from indigestion. For nausea and vomiting, two cardamoms should be taken, of which one should be roasted. Both cardamoms should be ground with a little water and taken as a drink.

• Foul smell

The aromatic flavour in cardamom is a good mouth cleaner. A few seeds chewed for a brief period will remove foul smell.

• Genito-urinary disorders

Cardamom helps increase the secretion and discharge of urine. It's powdered seeds, mixed with a tablespoon of banana leaf and Indian goosebery (amala) juice, taken thrice a day, serve as a valuable diuretic food. It is very effective in treating diseases like gonorrhoea, cystitis, nephritis, burning micturition or urination and scanty urination.

• Sexual dysfunctions

Cardamom is a sex stimulating food. It's use has been found beneficial in the treatment of sexual dysfunction like impotency and premature ejaculation. A pinch of powdered cardamom seeds, boiled in milk and sweetened with honey, should be taken every night. It will increase sexual stamina and virility. Excessive use of cardamom should, however, be avoided as it may have adverse effect.

• Depression

This spice is a mood elevating food and a decoction prepared from it has been found valuable in overcoming depression. This decoction is prepared by powdering the seeds and boiling them in water. It should be taken mixed with honey. It has a very pleasant aroma and it helps lift moods in case of depression.

• Hiccup

The use of cardamom has been found beneficial in the treatment of hiccup. An infusion should be prepared by boiling a couple of pounded whole cardamoms in a cup of water along with five leaves of mint. This infusion should be taken to releive the condition.

• Oral disorders

This spice has also been found beneficial in the treatment of pharyngitis, sore-throat, relaxed uvula and hoarseness during the infective stage of influenza. A gargle should be prepared from cardamom seeds and cinnamon and used in treating these conditions. This gargle used daily can protect a person against influenza virus.

• Headache

This spice has been found beneficial in the treatment of headache. It should be ground to a fine powder, and this powder should be used as a snuff to obtain relief.

• Kidney stones

The use of cardamom has been found valuable in kidney and bladder stones. The seeds should be consumed with the seeds of cucumber to obtain relief.

Uses

In India, cardamoms are used as masticatory and are often included in the betel quid. They are used for flavouring curries, cakes, bread and for other culinary purposes. Substantial quantities are imported into the Middle East, where they are used for flavouring coffee, meat dishes and sweetmeats. In Sweden and Finland, they are widely used in confectionery. The Americans use this spice in baked foods and the Russians in cakes and confectionery. The essential oil of cardamom is used both in pharmacy and perfumery, for flavouring liquors and bitters, in the preparation of tincture and as a stimulant.

Celery Seeds

A Tonic and Stimulant Food

7

Description

The celery *(Apium graveolens)* is an important salad plant, which grows upto a height of 60 to 180 cm. It consists of the bulbous roots, conspicuously joint stems and well developed green leaves, which emanate directly from the fleshy roots. The leaves are compound, with long stalk, which are big and succulent. The fruits are small in size, dark brown in colour and emanate a peculiar flavour when cut open. The seeds are brown in colour.

In India the leaves are not so popular, but the root and the seeds are commonly used in Unani and Ayurvedic medicine. The seeds are exported to European countries as condiments. It is mostly grown in kitchen or home gardens as a salad crop.

Origin and distribution

Celery is a native of Europe and Asia. It was known to Chinese in the fifth century. The Chinese plants are, however, of Asiatic origin, while those cultivated in Europe and America are derived from European plants.

In early days celery was not cultivated but it's leaves were collected for medicinal purposes. In England, where it grows wild, it was known as smallage and used in medicines. In the 16th and 17th centuries, it was brought into gardens and grown first as a medicinal plant and later as a flavouring for soups and stews. It is now grown widely in temperate regions and in the mountains of the tropics.

In India, large areas in Punjab and Uttar Pradesh are utilised for the cultivation of celery for the production of the seed. It grows best when the weather is relatively cool, with a well distributed moderate rainfall during the season. Elevation of over 3,000 ft are most suitable for its satisfactory growth.

Nutritive value/Composition

An analysis of celery seeds shows them to consist of moisture 5.1 percent, protein 18.1 percent, fat 22.8 percent, crude fibre 2.9 percent, carbohydrates 40.9 percent and total ash 10.2 percent per 100 gms. Their mineral and vitamin contents are calcium 1.8 percent, phosphorus 0.55 percent, iron 0.45 percent, sodium 0.17 percent, potassium 1.4 percent, thiamine 0.41 mg. percent, riboflavin 0.49 mg. percent, niacin 4.4 mg. percent, vitamin C 17.2 mg. percent and vitamin A 650 International units per 100 gms. Their calorific value is 450.

The celery leaves are the best sources of mineral salts and vitamins. An analysis of celery leaves shows them to consist of moisture 88.0 percent, protein 6.3 percent, fats 0.6 percent and carbohydrates 1.6 percent per 100 gms. Their mineral and vitamin contents are calcium 230 mg. percent, phosphorus 140 mg. percent, iron 6.3 mg. percent, carotene 3990 mg. percent, riboflavin 0.11 mg. percent, niacin 1.2 mg. percent and vitamin C 62 mg. percent. Their calorific value is 37.

The celery fuirts yield 2-3 percent of a pale yellow volatile oil with a persistent odour, characteristic of the plant. In trade, this is known as celery seed oil and is much valued both as a fixative and as an ingredient of perfumes. The principle constituents of this oil are d-limonene 60 percent, d-selinene 10 percent, 3 percent. The last two constituents are responsible for the aroma of the oil.

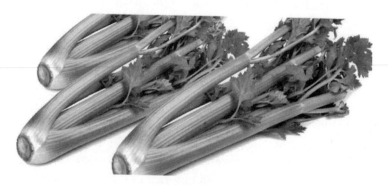

Celery seeds are carminative, diuretic and aphrodisiac.

Medicinal virtues

The word celery is derived from the Latin, celeri which means quick acting, and presumably refers to its therapeutic properties. The seeds, green leaves and stem are all extremely rich in active ingredient that make celery a very important medicinal plant. It has a well-balanced content of the basic minerals, vitamins and other nutrients, in addition, it has important concentration of plant hormones and the essential oils that gives celery its strong and characteristic smell. Besides having specific effect on the regulation of the nervous system, it also has a calming influence.

The seeds of celery relieve flatulence, increase the secretion and discharge of urine and promote sexual desire. They act as a tonic, laxative and stimulant. They are useful in counteracting spasmodic disorders and in promoting abortion. Recent discoveries by scientists reveal that celery seeds may afford protection against cancer, high blood pressure and high cholesterol.

• Rheumatism and gout

The alkaline elements in the celery greatly outweighs acidic elements. It is therefore effective in diseases resulting from acidity and toxemia. It is specially helpful in rheumatism and gout. A fluid extract of the seeds should be used to treat these conditions.

• Cancer

In a study for the National Cancer Institute, Luk Lam, Ph.D., and his colleagues at LKT Laboratories in St. Paul, Minnesota, have been analyzing the chemical constituents of celery seed oil and their effect on living beings. They isolated five compounds of interest and the compound senanolide was found to be most active. This and related compound butyl phthalide reduced the incidence of tumors in laboratory animals anywhere from 38 percent to 57 percent. The use of celery seeds can thus help prevent cancer.

• High-blood pressure

According to William J.Elliott, a   pharmacologist at the University of Chicago's Pritzker School of Medicine, celery has been used as a folk remedy, from 200 B.C, to lower blood pressure. He isolated a blood-pressure-reducing drug in celery. This chemical is, known as 3-n-butylphthalide, found in celery seed oil which gives aroma to the celery. Dr. Elliott says celery may be unique, because "the active blood-pressure lowering compound is found in rather high concentrations in celery". The person suffering from this disease should take two to four stalks.

As an alternative, the patient may take a tea made from the

celery seeds. This tea is prepared by pouring boiling water over one teaspoon of freshly crushed seeds. The seeds may be allowed to steep for 10 to 20 minutes before drinking.

• Nervous afflictions

Celery seeds are highly beneficial in the treatment of nervous afflictions resulting from degeneration of the sheathing of the nerves. They help to restore these to their normal conditions and thus alleviate the affliction. A tea made from the seeds may be used to treat these conditions in the same manner as for high blood pressure.

• Respiratory system disorders

Celery seeds are known to have anti-spasmodic properties. They are thus useful in the treatment of asthma, bronchitis, pleurisy and tuberculosis of lungs. For better results, a teaspoon of the seeds should be soaked in a cup of fenugreek seeds decoction and taken mixed with a tablespoon of honey every night. This treatment should be continued for a month.

• Indigestion

The seeds of celery are useful in indigestion. A teaspoon of the seeds soaked in a glass of buttermilk for five to six hours should be grounded in the same buttermilk mixture and given as a medicine to treat this conditions.

• Weakness and malnutrition

The powder of the dry root of the herb is a valuable tonic in general weakness and malnutrition. One teaspoon of this powder mixed with a tablespoon of honey should be taken twice daily in the treatment of these conditions. It restores the normal functioning of the disordered system.

• Insomnia

Celery leaves are useful in sleeplessness. The juice of the leaves, mixed with a tablespoon of honey, should be taken at night before retiring. It will help one to relax and sleep.

Uses

Celery seeds are used as spice. They are used for flavoring soups, stews and salad dressings. The seed oil is one of the most valuable flavouring agents as it imparts a warm, aromatic and pleasing flavour to food products. It is employed for flavouring different kinds of foods like canned soups, meats, sausages and particularly in the flavouring of the popular celery salts, celery tonic and culinary sauces. Celery leaves can be eaten either raw in salads form with other vegetables or in cooked form. Soup and juice can also be prepared from them.

Chillies or Capsicums

A Decongestant and Digestive Spice

8

Description

Chillies *(Capsicum annum)* are the dried ripe fruits of the species of genus capsicum. They are also called red peppers or capsicums. They are virtually an indispensable item for cooking. Dry chilli contributes a major share among the spices consumed per head in India.

Capsicum is a variable annual subshrub it has a single flower and usually pendent fruits. The fruits are long or oval having bright dark green colour and begin to change into beautiful crimson red on ripening. The fruits are broader at the base and conical at the tip. They grow from 2.5 to 15 cm. The pericap of the fruits consists of parenchymatous cells which contain droplets of red oil and have thin cellulose walls. The small fruited kinds are hot and pungent and the large fruited ones are generally mild.

Origin and distribution

Chilli plants are the native of America. Columbus in 1492 A.D. brought chilli on his first voyage back from America. Then the chilli spread along the Mediterranean coast and in

India, it was introduced by Portuguese in Goa. In Portuguese language chilli is called Maris. Chilli plants are mostly cultivated in South India. There are number of varieties that are used daily in culinary preparations.

Nutritive value/Composition

An analysis of green chilli shows it to consist of moisture 85.7 percent, protein 2.9 percent, fat 0.6 percent, fibre 6.8 percent and carbohydrates 3.0 percent. It's mineral and vitamin contentare calcium 30 mg. percent, phosphorous 80 mg. percent, iron 4.4 mg. percent, carotene 175 meg. percent, thiamine 0.19 mg. percent, riboflavin 0.39 mg. percent, niacin 0.9 mg. percent and vitamin C 111 mg. percent. Its calorific value is 29. An analysis of dry chilli shows it to consist of moisture 10.0 percent, protein 15.9 percent, fat 6.2 percent, fibre 30.2 percent, carbohydrates 31.6 percent. Its mineral and vitamin content are calcium 160 mg. percent, phosphorous 370 mg. percent, iron 2.3 mg.percent, carotene 345 mg. percent, thiamine 0.93 mg. percent, riboflavin 0.43 mg. percent, niacin 9.5 mg. percent and vitamin C 50 mg. percent. Its calorific value is 246.

The chief constituent of pericarp is a crystalline colourless, pungent principle known as Capsiacin or Capsicutin. It is secreted by the outerwalls of the fruit and occurs chiefly in the dissepiment which divides the fruit into two cavities. It's melting point is 63°C. When the fruits are burnt they emit an extremely irritable vapour which causes nasal and throat irritation. The fruits contain a fixed oil, red colouring matter which is not pungent and yield 20 to 25 percent of alcoholic extract. The seeds are bland contain some traces of starch. Green chillies are rich in Rutin.

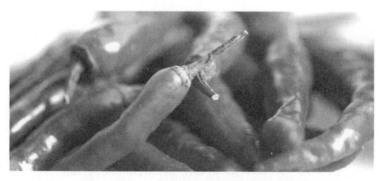

Hot chilli peppers are a powerful anti-coagulant food.

Medicinal virtues

Chillies are pungent and hot. Taken in moderation, they are useful as a decongestant and digestive. They strengthen the blood-clot-dissolving system, open up sinuses and air passages, break up mucus in the lungs, act as an expectorant or decongestant, and help prevent bronchitis and emphysema. Most of chilli pepper's pharmacological activity is credited to capsaicin, the compound that makes pepper taste hot. Capsaicin is also a potent painkiller, alleviating headaches when inhaled, and joint pain when injected. It also has antibacterial and antioxidant activity. Putting hot chilli sauce on food speeds up metabolism, burning off calories. Contrary to popular belief, chilli peppers do not harm the stomach lining or promote ulcers.

• Blood clots

Hot chilli peppers are a powerful anti-coagulant food. They are very effective in preventing blood clots. This evidence comes from Thailand, where people eat capsicum chilli peppers as a seasoning and as an appetizer. This infuses their blood with chilli pepper compounds several times a day. Research scientists believe that this may be a primary reason why thrombolisms, life-threatening blood clots, are rare among Thais.

To prove the theory, hematologist Sukon Visudhiphan, M.D., and colleagues at the Siriraj Hospital in Bangkok conducted a test. They fortified homemade rice noodles with hot pepper, using two teaspoons of fresh ground capsicum pepper in every 200 grams of noodles. Then they fed the peppery noodles to 16 healthy medical students. Four others ate plain noodles. Almost immediately, the clot-dissolving activity of the blood of the eaters of pepper-laced noodles rose but returned to normal in about 30 minutes. While nothing happened to the blood of the plain noodle eaters.

The effect of chilli pepper was thus short-lived. However, Dr. Visudhiphan believes that frequent stimulation through hot chillies continually clears the blood of clots. This makes Thai people generally less vulnerable to blockage of arteries.

• Depression

Hot chilli pepper is a mood elevating food and therefore beneficial in the treatment of depression. Its use can give a person a thrill that is more than purely sensory. According to Dr. Paul Rozin, a psychologist at the University of Pennsylvania, who has done extensive research on reactions to hot peppers, Capsaicin, the hot substance present in it can induce a rush of endorphins in the brain which can temporarily elevate mood.

Dr. Rozin explains that when a person eats, hot chillies, the capsaicin "burns" the nerve endings of the tongue and mouth, causing them to send false pain signals to the brain. In response, the brain tries to protect the body from perceived injury by secreting natural painkillers or endorphins. This lifts the mood and the person experiences a sense of well-being.

• Respiratory diseases

Hot chilli pepper is the best mucokinetic food among all hot spicy food. According to Dr. Irwin Ziment, M.D., professor of Medicine at UCLA, since antiquity, the flavoured foods for treating pulmonary and respiratory diseases have been mustard, garlic and hot chilli peppers. The active agents in these foods may work by several mechanisms. However, Dr. Ziment, believes that they generally activate a flash flood of fluids in air passages that thin out mucus, so that it flows more easily.

Dr. Ziment advises those who already suffer from chronic bronchitis and emphysema to eat hot food regularly, at least three times a week. He says that his patients who do so breathe more easily and require less treatment. Further, in surveys, he finds that those who eat more hot spicy cuisine are less likely to develop chronic bronchitis and emphysema, even if they smoke.

• Loss of hair

The use of red chillies have been found useful in preventing loss of hair and in promoting hair growth. Capsaicin in the chillies acts like canthridine. Red chillies may be boiled in Coconut Oil at the rate of 1 chilli per 120 ml. of oil. This oil should be applied to the hair. Its regular use increases hair growth and keeps them soft.

• Aches and pain

Capsaicin contained in the chillies suppresses pain by draining nerve cells of something called substance P, which relays pain sensations to the central nervous system. Thus, capsaicin helps block the perception of pain. Recently, the hot pepper essence has been injected or made into medications to help several diseases characterised by pain.

Concentrated chilli oil, prepared by roasting 4 chillies in 30 ml. of castor oil, makes a useful analgesic balm. This oil can be used beneficially in the treatment of rheumatic pains, sciatica and bursitis. Its regular application may cause blisters. Therefore, it should be carefully used. Capsicum liniments, tinctures, plasters are officially approved. These ointment contain capsaicin. They are useful analgesic balm.

Uses

The large fruited capsicums, which are generally mild, are used as vegetable. They are cooked like brinjals or stuffed with minced meat. The small kinds, which are hot and pungent, are used more as a condiment. Raw green chillies are used in the preparation of curries, pickles and they impart flavour. They are also used in vegetable salads to increase hunger. Powder of dry chillies is used in the preparation of condiments, pickles and curries.

Precaution

Chillies, especially in raw form, should not be consumed in excess, as their excessive use may induce labour in pregnant women and cause miscarriage. Excessive use of chillies causes diarrhoea and intense pain in the rectum, therefore, chillies should not be given to those who are not used to chilli preparations. The use of chillies should also be avoided in hyperacidity, stomatitis, gastric ulcer, hepatitis, anal fissure, bleeding piles, cystisis and nephritis.

Cinnamon

9

A Preventive against Nervous Tension

Description

The cinnamon *(Cinnamomum zeylanicum)* is an evergreen perennial tree, which grows upto a height of about 6 to 8 m. The leaves of the plant are large, 10 to 20 cm. in length and 6 to 10 cm. in width. They are egg-shaped, thick, leathery, pointed at tip and shining green and lighter coloured beneath. The flowers are minute, in large hairy clusters. Fruits are oblong or egg-shaped, about 1.5 to 2 cm. long and dark purple, with one seed.

The bark of the tree is thick, smooth and brownish dark in colour. The inner bark is obtained from carefully selected shoots. It is then cured and dried. During drying, the bark shrinks and curls into a cylinder or "quill". They have a pleasing fragrant odour and a warm, sweet and aromatic taste.

The shoots of the two year old cinnamon tree are cut and the bark is peeled after the branches are exposed to air for about twenty four hours. Then the bark is packed inside one another and dried. Cinnamon occurs in long cylindrical dry bark of brown colour. The bark is thin and brittle.

Cinnamon bark is one of the most popular spices used in every home. It has a delicate fragrance and a warm agreeable taste. It is extensively used as a spice or condiment in the form of small pieces or powder.

Origin and distribution

Cinnamon is a native of Sri Lanka and other parts of tropical Asia. It has been cultivated from very ancient times. Ancient Chinese herbals mention it as early as 2700 B.C. Cinnamon was an ingredient in ancient Egyptian embalming mixtures. In the Bible, Moses used it in holy anointing oil.

After the fall of Rome, trade between Europe and Asia became difficult, but cinnamon was so prized that it still found its way west.

A native of South India this tree occurs upto an altitude of about 1500, but is more common at lower altitudes, even below 200 m. It is also cultivated in certain parts of India. Today, Sri Lanka exports cinnamon to all parts of the world.

Nutritive value/Composition

An analysis of cinnamon shows it consist of moisture 9.9 percent, protein 4.6 percent, fat (ether extract) 2.2 percent, fibre 20.3 percent , carbohydrates 59.5 percent and total ash 3.5 percent per 100 gm. Its mineral and vitamin contents are calcium 1.6 percent, phosphorus 0.05 percent, iron 0.004 percent, sodium 0.01 percent, potassium 0.4 percent, thiamine 0.14 mg. percent, riboflavin 0.21 mg. percent, niacin 1.9 mg. percent, vitamin C 39.8 mg. percent and vitamin A 175 I.U., per 100 grams. Its calorific value is 355.

Cinnamon contains 2.0 percent of an essential oil known as cinnamon oil. This oil consists of 70-90 percent of eugenol. The bark contains 0.5-1.0 percent oil and green leaves yield about 1 percent oil. The root bark yields 3 percent oil, which differs from constituents of cinnamon oil are cinnamic aldehyde, eugenol, phellandrene and other terpenes.

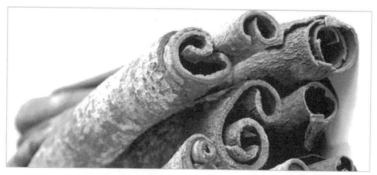

Cinnamon soothes stomach, controls blood sugar and prevents stomach ulcers.

Medicinal virtues

The Chinese used the bark of this tree as a medicine and Chinese herbalists still recommend it for fever, diarrhoea and menstrual problems. The Romans also knew about the medicinal value of this bark. Even Indians knew about the therapeutic uses of this herb long before the 8th century. The oldest record available about the description of cinnamon is in the Torah. The Ceylonese started collecting the bark of this tree for its medicinal use in the 12th century. It was, however, Khizvenee who was the first person to give details about the medicinal virtues of this herb in the 13th century.

The leaves can be used in the form of powder or decoction. They are stimulant and are useful in relieving flatulence and increasing secretion and discharge of urine. Cinnamon prevents nervous tension, improves complexion and memory. A pinch of cinnamon powder mixed with honey should be taken regularly every night for these conditions.

Cinnamon also soothes stomach incase of indigestion, controls blood sugar in diabetics, prevents stomach ulcers, wards off urinary tract infections, fights tooth decay and gum disease and prevents vaginal yeast infections. It gives a sweetish tingling warm feeling when chewed. It is astringent in taste.

• Infectious diseases

According to Daniel B. Mowrey, Ph.D., director of the American Phytotherapy Research Laboratory in Salt Lake City, Utah, and author of The Scientific Validation of Herbal Medicine, "Cinnamon is an antiseptic that helps kill bacteria that cause tooth decay and gum disease." Cinnamon also kills many disease causing fungi and viruses. One German study showed it "suppresses completely" the cause of most urinary tract infections and the fungus responsible for vaginal yeast infections.

• Viral diseases

Cinnamon is an antiviral food and is useful in preventing and treating viral infections. A drink made from it has disinfectant properties. This drink is prepared by putting half a teaspoon of tincture, obtained from the bark of cinnamon tree, in 285 ml of hot water. Taken daily before going into crowded places, it protects against colds and influenza, when these diseases are prevalent in an epidemic form. It also gives a glow of warmth to the whole body.

Cinnamon is also an effective remedy for cold and other viral infections when they have already occurred. A decoction should be prepared by boiling 5 cm. of coarsely powdered cinnamon in a glass of water with a pinch of pepper powder and honey. This decoction can be beneficially used as a medicine in case of influenza, sore throat and malaria. Cinnamon oil, mixed with honey, also gives immense relief from cold.

• Chronic indigestion

Cinnamon stimulates digestion and relieves gas in the stomach. It should be used in the form of decoction in the same manner as for cold and influenza. This decoction can also be used as a carminative medicine for flatulence and indigestion. A tablespoon of this water should be taken half an hour after meals. Cinnamon also checks nausea, vomiting and diarrhoea. Cinnamon oil 1 to 2 drops taken on a lump of sugar thrice daily also acts as a carminative-antiseptic medicine for indigestion, diarrhoea, flatulent colic and dyspepsia.

• Diabetes

Cinnamon appears to help people with diabetes metabolize sugar. In non-insulin-dependent type of diabetes, the pancreas produces insulin, but the body cannot use it efficiently to break down glucose, the simple sugar that fuels body functions. U.S. Department of Agriculture (USDA) researchers discovered that cinnamon reduces the amount of insulin necessary for glucose metabolism.

"One-eighth of a teaspoon of cinnamon triples insulin efficiency," says James A. Duke, Ph.D., a botanist retired from the USDA and author of The CRC Handbook of Medicinal Herbs. For people with diabetes, 1/8 to 1/4 teaspoon of ground cinnamon per meal may help control blood sugar levels.

• Natural birth-control

This spice can be used as a natural birth-control. It has a remarkable effect on checking the early release of ova after child-birth. A piece of cinnamon taken every night after a month of child-birth thus delays menstruation for more than 15 to 20 months and prevents early conception. It also indirectly helps the secretion of breast milk and it has been proved that prolonged breast feeding checks the appearance of menstruation after child-birth.

• Women's problems

The use of cinnamon has been found valuable in reducing labour pain during child-birth. A decoction of this spice should be taken in treating this condition.

• Headache

The headache produced by exposure to cold air is readily removed by plastering the temples and the forehead with a paste of finely powdered cinnamon in water. Rubbing the forehead with cinnamon oil also relieves headache.

• Toothache

The oil of cinnamon has been found beneficial in the treatment of toothache. A cotton swab should be drenched with one or two drops of the oil and placed on a painful tooth to obtain relief.

• Acne

The use of cinnamon has been found beneficial in the treatment of Acne. A paste should be prepared from powdered cinnamon with few drops of fresh lime juice. This paste can be applied beneficially over pimples and blackheads.

• Other ailments

Cinnamon is beneficial in the treatment of several other ailments, including spasmodic afflictions, asthma, paralysis, excessive menstruation, uterus disorders and gonorrhoea. The aromatic flavour of cinnamon is good mouth cleaner. It removes the foul smell. A pinch of cinnamon powder taken with honey, daily at night, helps stop frequent passing of urine during the day.

Uses

Dried Cinnamon leaves and inner bark are used for flavouring cakes, sweets and in curry powder. They are also used in incense, dentrifrices and perfumes. Cinnamon bark oil is used for flavoring confectionery and liqueurs and in pharmaceutical and dental preparations. Cinnamon leaf oil is used in perfumes and flavorings and also in the synthesis of vanillin. Cinnamon oil is found to be an excellent food preservative.

Precaution

The excessive use of cinnamon should be avoided as it may prove harmful to the kidneys and the bladder. Pregnant women should avoid the use of this spice, as it may bring about abortion. Persons of hot constitution should also avoid its use, as it may cause headache in them.

Clove

A Spice for Youthful Digestion

10

Description

The clove *(Syzyigium aromaticum)* tree is a middle-sized, evergreen tree. It has a straight trunk and grows upto a height of 10 to 12 meters. Cloves are dried buds of this tree. The buds are collected when they develop a crimson color. When dried, they change into dark reddish-brown color. Each bud measures about 1.25 cm long. In India, clove trees are mostly grown in Kerala and Tamil Nadu.

The word clove is derived from the French word 'clov' and the English word 'clout', both of which means nail. It resembles a broad-headed nail. It is one of the most valuable spices of the Orient.

Origin and distribution

Clove has been used in India and China from ancient times, both as a spice and medicine to check tooth decay and bad breath. Charaka, the great ancient medical authority, has mentioned the carminative value of this spice. In Persia and China it was credited with aphrodisiac property.

Nutritive value/Composition

An analysis of the dry clove shows it to consist of moisture

25.2 percent, protein 5.2 percent, fat 8.9 percent, minerals 5.2 percent, fibre 9.5 percent and carbohydrates 46.0 percent per 100 grams.

Its mineral and vitamin contents are calcium 740 mg percent, phosphorous 100 mg percent, iron 11.7 mg percent, carotene 253 meg percent, Thiamine 0.08 mg percent and riboflavin 0.13 mg percent. Its calorific value is 286.

The clove buds, stem and leaves, on steam distillation, yield a substantial amount of essential oil. The clove bud oil, derived from the dried buds on steam distillation, contains free eugenol, eugenol acetate and caryophyllene. The oil from the stem contains more eugenol than the oil from the bud, besides eugenol acetate, in a small quantity. The leaf oil contains much less of total eugenol than the bud oil and a very small quantity of eugenol acetate and caryophyllene.

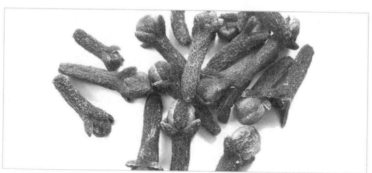

Cloves helps stimulate sluggish circulation and promote youthful digestion.

Medicinal virtues

Clove has many medicinal properties. These properties emanate from volatile oil contained in it. This oil is stimulant, carminative, antiseptic, antispasmodic and expectorant. It also helps stimulate sluggish circulation and thereby promote youthful digestion and metabolism.

In the Indian system of medicine, cloves are used in various conditions either in the form of a powder or a decoction made from them. Clove oil contains ingredients that help stabilise blood circulation and regulate body temperature. This oil, applied outwardly, has stimulating effects on the skin, producing heat and redness.

• Digestive Disorders

This spice is of great value as a gas relieving food. It is highly beneficial in the treatment of several digestive disorders like indigestion and flatulent colic. A decoction is prepared by boiling 6 cloves in 30 ml of water. This decoction should be taken thrice daily after meals as a carminative medicine in treating these conditions. A drop or two of clove oil on a lump of sugar and pinch of soda-bicarb can also be taken thrice daily with beneficial results for the same purpose.

Licking the powder of fried cloves, mixed with honey, is effective in controlling vomiting. The anaesthetic action of clove numbs the gullet and stomach and stops vomiting. In case of acute diarrhoea and vomiting caused by food poisoning, six cloves should be put in a glass of water and allowed to stand for 12 hours. A tablespoon of malt vinegar and a pinch of salt should be added to this water and stirred well. It should be given to the patient in doses of one teaspoon every half an hour.

• Aches and pains

Clove is of great value as a pain killing spice. It has long been used to kill pain in toothache. A clove or cotton dipped in clove oil placed in the cavity caused by dental caries, stops pain and prevents the accumulation of food particles in them. A clove sauted in a teaspoon of sesame oil and 3 to 5 drops of this warm oil put into the ear can cure earache.

Muscular cramps are often relieved when the oil of clove is applied as a poultice on the affected part. In painful condition of joints, neuralgia and migraine, five drops of clove oil, mixed in 30ml of olive oil, can be applied as a liniment with beneficial result.

A paste of clove and salt crystals in milk is a common household remedy for headaches. While clove helps reduce pain, salt as a hygroscopic agent, absorbs fluid and decreases tension.

• Infections

Clove is an antibacterial food and it helps fight infections. Its use in case of toothache decreases infection, besides reducing pain. Cloves are also effective in treating cholera infection. About four grams of this spice should be boiled in three litres of water until half the water has evaporated. This water, taken during draughts, will check severe symptoms of the disease.

• Rheumatic affliction

This popular spice is an anti-inflammatory food. It has long been used to treat arthritis and other rheumatic diseases. This property emanates from its main ingredient eugenol. Clove brings relief mainly by blocking formation of hormone-like substance that induce inflammation. A clove may be chewed twice daily in treating these conditions.

• Prevents blood clots

This spice is a powerful anti-coagulant food. It helps keep the blood free of dangerous clots. According to Dr. Krishna Srivastava of Odense Univerity in Denmark, cloves are stronger than aspirin in this respect. The primary active agent in this spice eugenol, also helps protect the structure of platelets even after they have been aggregated. Cloves help reduce the production of thromboxane, which is a powerful promoter of platelet clumping.

• Respiratory disorders

Clove possesses mucus-clearing property. It is thus an effective remedy for respiratory disorders like asthma and bronchitis. A teaspoon of decoction, prepared by boiling 6 cloves in 30 ml of water, makes an excellent expectorant medicine. It should be taken with honey three times daily for treating these conditions.

To alleviate the spasms of painful cough in tuberculosis, asthma and bronchitis, 3 to 5 drops of clove oil, mixed with honey and a clove of garlic, should be taken before going to bed.

Clove oil, mixed with a little turpentine, can also be beneficially massaged over the chest in bronchitis, pneumonia and whooping cough.

In pharyngitis, chewing a clove with a crystal of common salt eases expectoration, relieves the irritation in the throat and stops cough. Chewing a burnt clove is also effective remedy for cough caused by relaxed throat and pharyngitis.

• Stye

Clove is one of the best remedies for styes, which is an inflammation around the eyelash. A clove stub rubbed in water and then applied over the stye gives relief.

• Sexual debility

Clove is an aphrodisiac food and its use has been found beneficial in the treatment of sexual weakness and debility. A hole should be made in moringa tree, which is a variety of drumstick tree grown in South India. As many cloves as possible should be inserted in this hole, which should then be closed with wax. The cloves so placed should be removed after 40 days, dried in shade and kept in an airtight bottle.

Holding one such clove under the tongue after eating during the sexual intercourse, prolongs the act by controlling the ejaculatory centers in the brain and gives immense pleasure during ejaculation. Eating such cloves daily once with a half boiled egg and a tablespoon of honey regularly, increases sexual strength and potency.

Uses

Cloves are used as a table spice and mixed with chillies, cinnamon, turmeric and other spices in the preparation of curry powder. They are also used to flavour the betel quid (paan). Clove oil is used in the manufacture of perfumes, soaps, bath salts and as a flavouring agent in medicine and dentistry.

Coriander

11

Valuable in spasmodic Disorders

Description

The coriander *(Coriandrum sativum)*, is a well-known condiment crop. It abounds in season by the fascinating bunchful in almost every vegetable shop. Fresh coriander leaves and dried coriander seeds are used almost daily in Indian homes in scores of curries and other vegetable preparations.

This plant is both annual and perennial. It is an erect and sweet smelling plant and grows up to 20 cm. in length with many branches. The stem is very feeble, smooth and light green in colour. Leaves are compound, very thin, alternate and easily breakable. The flowers found in branched umbels are very small, white or pinkish.

The fruits of the plant are spherical, about one centimetre in diameter, with some longitudinal ridges. They are green in colour when tender and are brownish yellow, when they are ripened. They have a sweet smelling fragrance when they are fresh. Practically all the parts of the plant, that is, tender stem, the leaves, flowers and the fruits have a pleasant aromatic odour.

Coriander seeds are dry when they are ripe. The seeds consist of two firmly united mericarps and look globular. They are brownish-yellow in colour and measure about 5 mm. in diameter. On each half of the seed there are five wavy ridges. Seeds are smooth and are crowned with the remains of calyx teeth and styles. They have an aromatic odour and agreeable spicy taste. Powder of the roasted coriander seeds is blended with other spices to prepare condiments since ancient times in India, Rome, Iran and Arabia.

Origin and distribution

The coriander is native to Mediterranean Europe and western Asia. The Egyptians used it centuries ago. Hippocrates and other Greek physicians employed it in their medicines. The Romans first introduced coriander to Britian, where it is now established as an indigenous plant. It has been naturalized in North America.

Coriander is now extensively cultivated in Europe, North Africa, India, South America, Malaysia, Thailand and China. It has been introduced into several tropical countries. In India, it is cultivated practically in all the states. It thrives in black soil and arid regions.

Nutritive value/Composition

Coriander is rich in various food elements. An analysis of coriander leaves shows them to contain moisture 86.3 percent, protein 3.3 percent, fat 0.6 percent, minerals 2.3 percent, fibre 1.2 percent and carbohydrates 6.3 percent per 100 grams. Their mineral and vitamin contents include calcium 184 mg. percent, phosphorus 71 mg. percent, iron 18.5 mg. percent, carotene 6918 meg. percent, thiamine 0.05 mg. percent, riboflavin 0.06 mg. percent, niacin 0.8 mg. percent and vitamin C 135 mg. percent per 100 grams. They also contain 4 mgs. of sodium, 453 mgs. of potassium and 5 mgs. of oxalic acid per 100 grams. Their calorific value is 44.

An analysis of coriander seeds show them to contain moisture 11.2 percent, protein 14.1 percent, fat 16.1 percent, minerals 4.4 percent, fibre 32.6 percent and carbohydrates 21.6 percent vper 100 grams. Their mineral and vitamin contents are calcium 630 mg. percent, phosphorus 393 mg. percent, iron 17.9 mg. vpercent, corotene 942 meg. percent, thiamine 0.22 mg. per vcent, riboflavin 0.35 mg. percent and niacin 1.1 percent. Their calorific value is 288.

Coriander seeds contain volatile oil, which varies from 0.1 to 1.7 percent, depending upon the type of seed, soil and climate. Indian coriander oil is colourless, pale yellow liquid with characteristic odour and taste of coriander. The volatile oil is made up of hydrocarbons and oxygenated compounds. The hydrocarbons account for 20 percent of the essential oil. The major oxygenated compounds present are coriandrol and terpene-d-pinene 45 percent to 65 percent and 5 percent respectively. The oil causes irritation when in contact with skin for long time.

Medicinal virtues

Coriander was first introduced into Chinese medicine around 600 A.D. Galenical preparations of coriander seed have similar uses as a carminative, digestive, or stomachic in traditional Chinese, Indian, and Greco-European medicines. In Ayurvedic medicine it is usually combined with caraway and cardamom seeds, among others, while in European medicine it is usually combined with caraway, fennel and anise.

The leaves of coriander strengthen the stomach and promote its action. They relieve flatulence, increase secretion and discharge of urine and reduce fever. They promote sexual desire, help in the removal of catarrhal matters and phelgm from the bronchial tubes and counteract spasmodic disorders.

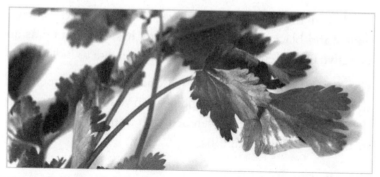

Coriander leaves relieve flatulence, increase the flow
of urine and reduce fever.

Coriander seeds are carminative, aromatic, antispasmodic and
stimulant. They reduce feverishness and promote a feeling of
coolness. Coriander juice is highly beneficial in deficiencies
of vitamins A, B1, B2, C and iron.

In Germany, coriander is used as a medicinal tea and a
component of carminative and laxative remedies, in
alcoholic distillate and drops dosage forms, often combined
with anise, caraway, or fennel. In the United States, coriander
is used as a carminative or digestive component of
compounds in confection, infusion, syrup and tincture dosage
forms. It is sometimes used in laxative compound preparations
to counteract or modify harsh stomach-upsetting effects.

• Digestive disorders

The juice of fresh coriander leaves is beneficial in the
treatment of digestive disorders such as indigestion, nausea,
piles, dysentery, hepatitis and ulcerative colitis. One or two
teaspoons of this juice should be taken mixed in fresh
buttermilk. It is also valuable in typhoid fever.

Dry coriander seeds have also been found valuable in
diarrhoea and chronic dysentery. They are also beneficial in
the treatment of piles, intestinal worms and acidity. A chutney

made from dry coriander seeds, green chillies, grated coconut, ginger and black grapes without seeds has been found as an effective home remedy for abdominal pain due to indigestion.

Coriander seeds are also beneficial in the treatment of dyspepsia, flatulent colic, indigestion and biliousness. A decoction of the seeds sweetened with honey should be used in treating these conditions.

• Small Pox

The use of fresh coriander juice has been found to be a valuable preventive. One teaspoon of this juice should be taken once daily, mixed with one or two seeds of banana, for seven days regularly. During actual infection of small pox, the juice of the fresh leaves should be instilled in the eyes. This will help prevent eye damage, which is common in this disease.

• High cholesterol levels

The dry seeds of coriander are powerful cholesterol lowering food. Their use has thus been found beneficial in the treatment of high blood cholesterol.

A decoction should be prepared by boiling two tablespoons of dry seeds in a glass of water. It should be cooled and strained. This decoction should be taken twice daily for few months. This will serve as a good diuretic and stimulate the kidneys, thereby bring down cholesterol level.

• Conjunctivitis

The use of freshly dried coriander seeds has been found beneficial in the treatment of conjunctivitis. A decoction should be prepared and used as an eye-wash in treating this condition. It will relieve burning, reduce pain and swelling.

• Excessive menstruation

Coriander seeds are beneficial in the treatment of excessive menstruation. Six grams of the seeds should be boiled in half litre of water, boil till there is half the quantity of water. Sugar candy should be added to it and the patient should drink it while it is still warm. It will bring relief after taking this medicine for three or four days.

• Sexual impotence

Coriander seeds are a powerful aphrodisiac food. Their use has thus been found valuable in sexual debility and impotence. Half a teaspoon of powder of the fresh roasted seeds mixed with honey makes an effective medicine for the treatment of spermatorrhoea and pre-mature ejaculation. It should be given once daily for a month.

• Skin disorders

A teaspoon of the juice extracted from the fresh leaves, mixed with a pinch of turmeric powder, is an effective remedy for pimples, blackheads and dry skin. The mixture should be applied on the face after thoroughly washing it, every night before retiring.

• Piles

The use of coriander seeds has been found valuable in piles. A strong decoction of the seeds should be prepared and taken with milk and jaggery or honey in treating this condition.

• Headache

The seeds are beneficial in the treatment of headache. They should be used in the form of poultice. It makes an effective cooling application.

Uses

The entire coriander plant, when young, is used for preparing chutneys and sauces. The fresh leaves are used for flavouring curries and soups. Chutneys can be made by mixing tomatoes or amla and coconut kernel with coriander leaves. The seeds are extensively employed as a condiment in the preparation of curry powder, pickling spices, sausages and seasoning. They are used for flavouring breads, cakes, pastries and cookies. A decoction made from dry seeds mixed with milk is used as a drink. Coriander seeds are generally used after mild roasting.

The seeds contain a volatile oil, which is used for flavouring and in medicine. It is used as a flavouring agent for spirituous liquors and in the cocoa and chocolate industries. It is also a valuable ingredient in perfumes. Decyldehyde (0.1% of volatile oil) is also useful in perfumery. Decyldehyde is obtained by treating the volatile oil with bisulphite.

Precautions

Dry coriander seeds should be sparingly used by persons suffering from bronchial asthma and chronic bronchitis, as they may aggravate the symptoms of these diseases.

Cumin Seeds

A Remedy for Digestive Disorders

12

Description

The cumin *(Cuminum cyminum)* plant belongs to the coriander family. It is one of the oldest spices, known since Biblical times. Cumin is an annual plant with a smooth surface and long slender and perpendicular root. It grows up to a height of 35-45 cm. It produces stems, arising almost from the base, with many branches. These branches bear leaves which are divided into long, narrow segments like Fennel, but much smaller and are of a deep green colour, generally turned back at the ends. The upper leaves are nearly stalkless, but the lower ones have longer leaf-stalks. The flowers are small, rose-coloured or white.

The plant has aromatic seed-like fruit, commonly known as 'cumin seed'. It is approximately 6 mm. long, oval in shape, and light yellowish-brown in colour. It has strong aromatic smell and warm, bitterish taste, which is due to the presence of a volatile oil.

Origin and distribution

Cumin plant is indeginous to upper Egypt, but it was cultivated from early times in Arabia, India, China and countries bordering the Mediterranean. It was used by Egyptians in 5000 B.C. both to season meats, fish, stews and to mummify their dead. The Romans used cumin as a substitute for pepper, and Pliny described it as the best appetizer of all seasonings.

In the Middle Ages, when cumin was very popular, Europeans believed it would keep poultry from wandering away, and even ensure fidelity between couples. The Germans carried cumin, dill and salt in their pockets when being wed, and in parts of Europe, a soldier would share a farewell wine powdered with cumin or carry with him a loaf of cumin bread baked by his sweetheart.

Cumin is now extensively grown in India, Iran, Morocco,China, Southern Russia, Indonesia, Japan and Turkey. It is cultivated in all the states of India except Assam and West Bengal. The chief producing centres are punjab and Uttar Pradesh.

Nutritive value/Composition

An anlaysis of cumin seeds shows them to consist of moisture 11.9 percent, protein 18.7 percent, fat 15.0 percent, crude fibre 12.0 percent, carbohydrates 36.6 percent and mineral matter 5.8 percent per 100 grams. Their mineral and vitamin contents are calcium 1080 mg. percent, phosphorous 511 mg. percent, iron 11.7 mg. percent, sodium 0.16 percent, potassium 2.1 percent, thiamine 0.55 mg. percent, riboflavin 0.36 mg. percent and niacin 2.6 mg. percent, vitamin C 3 mg. percent and vitamin A 175 I.U. per 100 grams. Their calorific value is 356.

On steam distillation, the crushed cumin seeds yield 2.5 percent to 4.5 percent of valuable volatile oil. This oil is pale-yellow in colour and turns dark on storage. The volatile oil contains cumin aldehyde, which is readily converted artificially into

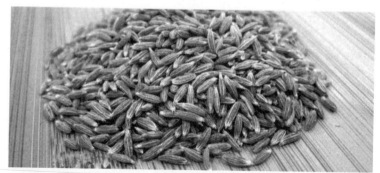

Cumin seeds are used for curing intestinal worms and is an antiseptic.

thymol. The other constituents of this oil are Thyme, cuminol, carvone, cynol and terpene.

Medicinal virtues

The fruit is a rich source of thymol, which is used as an anthelmintic against hookworm infections and also as an antiseptic. It forms part of many proprietary preparations. It is a stimulant. It increases the secretion and discharge of urine and relieves flatulence. It also strengthens the stomach and arrests bleeding.

• Digestive system disorders

Cumin seeds are highly beneficial in the treatment of several digestive system disorders such as biliousness, morning sickness, indigestion, atonic dyspepsia, diarrhoea in malabsorption syndrome, and flatulent colic. One teaspoon of cumin seeds should be boiled in a glass of water and the infusion should be mixed with one teaspoon of fresh coriander leaf juice and a pinch of salt. This preparation should be taken twice daily after meals as a medicine in treating these conditions.

Half a teaspoon of powdered cumin seeds, mixed in a teaspoon of tamarind pulp and honey is also a valuable remedy for morning sickness, jaundice, nausea, vomiting and bilious gidiness. This mixture should be licked before breakfast in treating these conditions. Chewing few seeds half an hour before food, increases hunger, and helps in digestion. Chewing the cumin seeds after food, prevents dental caries, indigestion, fermentation of food in the intestine and constipation.

Cumin water, is the water left over after the essential oil and thymol have been extracted by steam distillation. This water is commonly used in India as a carminative and is considered beneficial in the treatment of flatulence and griping, especially in children.

• Diarrhoea and dysentery

Cumin Seeds are valuable in diarrhoea and dysentery. A teaspoon or five grams of cumin seed powder should be taken with water three times daily in treating these conditions. Some jaggery or honey may be added to overcome its slight pungent taste.

• Piles

Black cumin seeds are valuable in piles. About 30 grams each of the roasted and unroasted seeds, should be ground together. Three grams of this mixture should be taken with water in treating this disease.

• Sleeplessness

Cumin seeds are a calming and sedative food. They soothe the nervous system and are thus valuable in sleeplessness. A teaspoon of the fried powder of cumin seeds should be mixed with the pulp of a ripe banana and taken as the last thing at night in the treatment of this condition.

• Cancer

Researchers in Israel and India are studying cumin's anticancer properties. In one series of tests, Indian scientists found that cumin increased the activity of a detoxifying body chemical (GST) that protects against certain kinds of cancer. At the Cancer Institute, Adyar, Chennai, cumin was found to block 83% of the chromosome damage that would normally be caused by a powerful cancer-causing chemical.

• Renal colic

Black cumin seeds are beneficial in the treatment of Renal colic. For better results, these seeds should be mixed with caraway seeds and black salt. This mixture, which should contain about 20 grams of cumin seeds, 12 grams of caraway seeds and six grams of black salt, should be ground together and mixed with little vinegar. Three grams of this mixture should be taken every hour till one feels better.

• Infections

Cumin seeds are powerful antibacterial food. The thymol contained in it is an anthelmintic against hookworm infections and also as an antiseptic in many proprietary preparations. A decoction prepared from cumin seeds is an antiseptic beverage and very useful in common colds and fever.

To prepare this decoction, a teaspoon of cumin seed is added to boiling water, which is allowed to simmer for a few seconds and set aside to cool. If the cold is associated with sore throat, a few small pieces of dry ginger should be added to this decoction. This soothes throat irritation.

• Sinusitis

Cumin seeds are also beneficial in the treatment of sinusitis. A teaspoon of these seeds should be tied in a thin cotton cloth and inhaled by the patient. It will give relief. The condition can also be relieved by taking a mixture of 100 grams of cumin seeds, fried and ground, alongwith 200 grams of pure honey.

• Pregnancy and lactation

A decoction of the cumin seeds mixed with milk and honey, used once daily during the entire period of pregnancy, helps the development of the baby and eases child-birth. It also increases the secretion of breast milk.

• Forgetfulness

This spice is a brain food. Its use has been found beneficial in the treatment of dullness of memory and forgetfulness. Three grams of powdered black cumin seeds mixed with 12 grams of pure honey can be licked in treating this condition.

• Boils

Black cumin seeds have been found beneficial in the treatment of boils. These seeds should be ground in water and applied as a paste over the affected parts.

• Scorpion sting

The paste of the cumin seeds has also proved valuable in scorpion sting. It should be prepared with onion juice and applied over the affected area.

• Bleeding

Cumin seeds are also beneficial in the treatment of bleeding from nose and lungs. An infusion of these seeds should be mixed with fresh lime juice and taken by the patient suffering from these problems.

Uses

Cumin seeds are extensively used in mixed spices and for flavoring curries, soups, sausages, bread and cakes. They are an ingredient of curry powder, pickles and chutneys. They are also used in Indian medicine.

Cumin oil is used in many types of flavouring preparations, particularly in curries and culinary preparations. In medicine, it is sometimes used as a carminative.

Curry Leaves

A Herbal Tonic

13

Description

The Curry tree *(Murraya Koenigii)* is a beautiful, aromatic more or less deciduous perennial shrub, which grows upto six metres in height. It is a small downy tree belonging to the orange family and is usually grown as a backyard tree. This evergreen tree has a small crooked round trunk about 15 to 30 cm diameter. The trunk is covered with greyish black bark. The tree has many arching branches with more foliages on the terminal twigs.

The leaves of this tree, called curry leaves, are divided into numerous leaflets. These leaflets are alternate, opposite, elliptic, sessile, smooth, thick, hard, strong and pungent. They have strong flavour because of the oil content present in the leaves. The leaves are about 3 to 5 cm. in length, with minutely toothed margin. They are slightly bitter and aromatic. The tree has numerous flowers, which are sweet scented, white and bell shaped. Berries are round, purplish black when ripe, and are found in bunches in the month of May.

Origin and distribution

A native of India and Sri Lanka, this grows in all tropical

zones and more so in rich soils. It is cultivated extensively for its aromatic leaves and ornamental value throughout India. It is commonly found in forests, often as gregarious undergrowth along the foot of the Himalayas from the Ravi to Sikkim and Assam. It is also found in West Bengal, Madhya Pradesh and in south and south-western states, namely, Maharashtra, Tamil Nadu, Kerala and Andhra Pradesh.

Nutritive value/Composition

An analysis of curry leaves shows them to consist moisture 63.8 percent, protein 6.1 percent, fat (ether extract) 1.0 percent, carbohydrates 18.7 percent, fibre 6.4 percent and mineral matter 4.0 percent per 100 grams. Their mineral and vitamin contents are calcium 830 mg percent, phosphorus 57 mg percent, iron 0.93 mg percent, Carotene 7,560 meg percent, Thiamine 0.08 mg percent, Riboflavin 0.21 mg percent, Niacin 2.3 mg percent and vitamin C 4 mg percent. Their calorific value is 108.

Fresh leaves on steam distillation under pressure yield 2.6 percent volatile oil. Rectified curry leaf oil is deep yellow in colour with a strong spicy odour and pungent clove-like taste. Besides the oil, the leaves contain a residual glucoside named as koenigin. The fruit yeilds 0.76 percent of yellow volatile oil. This oil has neroli like odour and pepper like taste, accompanied by an agreeable sensation of coolness on the tongue.

Medicinal virtues

Curry leaves possess the qualities of a herbal tonic. They strengthen the functions of stomach and promote its action. They are also used as a mild laxative. The leaves may be taken mixed with other mild tasting herbs. The juice extracted from 15 grams of leaves may be taken with buttermilk.

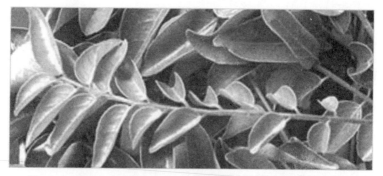

Curry leaves strengthen the stomach and are mild laxative.

• Digestive disorders

The curry leaves are valuable in digestive system disorders like morning sickness, nausea and vomiting due to indigestion and excessive use of fats. One or two teaspoons of fresh juice of the leaves, mixed with a teaspoon each of lime juice and honey, forms an effective medicine for treating these conditions. An infusion of the roasted leaves can be used beneficially to stop vomitting. The curry leaves, ground to a fine paste and mixed with buttermilk, can also be taken on an empty stomach in case of stomach upsets.

Tender curry leaves are also beneficial in the treatment of diarrhoea, dysentery and piles. They should be taken, mixed with honey. The bark of the tree is also valuable in bilious vomiting. A teaspoon of the powder or the decoction of the dry bark should be given with cold water in treating this condition.

• Diabetes

Curry leaves are an anti-diabetic food. Diabetes due to hereditary factors can be prevented by eating 10 fresh fully grown curry leaves every morning for three months. This has also been found beneficial in the treatment of diabetes due to obesity, as curry leaves possess weight reducing properties.

With the reduction in weight the patient stops passing sugar in urine.

• Kidney disorders

The root of the curry plant has been found valuable in relieving pain associated with the kidneys. The juice of the root can be taken in treating this condition.

• Premature greying of hair

Liberal intake of curry leaves have been found beneficial in the prevention and treatment of premature greying of hair. These leaves have the property to nourish the hair roots. New hair roots that grow are healthier with normal pigment. The leaves can be used in the form of chutney or the juice may be squeezed and taken in buttermilk or lassi.

When the leaves are boiled in coconut oil till they are reduced to a blackened residue, the oil forms an excellent hair tonic to stimulate hair growth and in retaining the natural pigmentation.

• Burns and Bruises

Curry leaves can be effectively used to treat burns, bruises and skin eruptions. They should be applied as a poultice over the affected areas.

• Eye disorders

Fresh juice of curry leaves instilled in the eyes makes them look bright. It also prevents the early development of cataract.

• Insect bites

The fruits of the tree, which are berries, are edible. They are green when raw, but purple when ripe. Juice of these berries, mixed with equal proportion of lime-juice, is an effective fluid for external application in insect stings and bites of poisonous creatures.

Uses

Curry leaves have been used for centuries in South India as a natural flavouring agent in *sambar, rasam* and *curries.* Chutney can be made by mixing the leaves with coriander leaves, coconut scrapings and tomatoes. The leaves, bark and the root of the curry plant are used in indigenous medicine.

Dill

14

A Soothing Spice

Description

Dill *(Anethum sowa)* is a green leafy vegetable and a culinary herb. It is both an annual and biennial plant with smooth surface, finely dissected light green leaves, small yellow flowers and elliptic, flattened fruits. The single stalks spring up to a height of one metre. Dill is derived from dilla which means to lull indicating its old reputation as a soothing herb.

The leaves are slightly pungent, aromatic and bitter in taste. They should be taken only mixed with other mild tasting leaves. About 30 ml. juice of the leaves can be taken with any other juice.

Origin and distribution

Dill is a native to the Mediteranean region, Southern Russia and Scandinavia. Over 3000 years ago, Dill was recorded in Egyptian hieroglyphics as a medicinal herb. The Romans brought it to England. It is now grown widely in Asia Minor, North Africa, India and in all other tropical countries. This plant is found practically all over India. It is also cultivated as a cold weather crop in many parts of the country.

The dill plant was known to the ancient Greeks and Romans.

It has been referred to in early saxon manuscripts and it was often mentioned by writers in the Middle ages. Greeks covered their heads with dill leaves so as to induce sleep. It was also considered a charm against witchcraft in the middle ages and was burned to drive away thunderous clouds and sulphurous fumes.

Nutritive value/Composition

An analysis of Indian dill shows it to consists of moisture 4.5 percent, mineral matter 5.89 percent to 11.54 percent, acid-in-soluble ash 0.55 percent to 2.71 percent and extraneous matter 3.16 percent to 12.93 percent per 100 grams.

The seeds of the plant yield 3 percent to 3.5 percent of an essential oil known as dill oil. The roots yield essential oil containing 95 percent of pinene. The spice yields 0.062 percent essential oil with high proportion of terpenes.

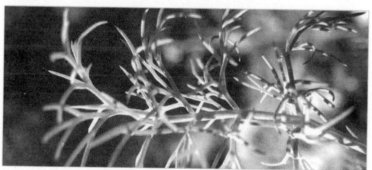

Dill leaves are calming and soothing medicine.

Medicinal virtues

Dill leaves are stimulant. They are useful in increasing secretion and discharge of urine and in counteracting spasmodic disorders. They are a soothing and calming medicine and help improve the functional activity of the stomach.

• Digestive system disorders

Dill helps settle the stomach, because it is a digestive aid. In fact, the ancient Egyptians, Greeks, Romans and Chinese all used it to soothe the stomach. Eating dill in its cooked form regularly aids digestion and prevents constipation. It is especially useful for children. One or two teaspoons of decoction of the fresh leaves mixed with each baby food will prevent digestive disorders in babies and help them sleep well.

A tea made from dill seeds is also considered benefical in the treatment of digestive disorder. To prepare this tea, two teaspoons of mashed seeds should be put in a cup of boiling water and steeped for ten minutes. This tea should be drunk up to three cups a day. To treat colic or gas in children under two, small amounts of a weak tea should be given.

The Dill oil, obtained by distillation of the seeds, is also an effective medicine for hyperacidity, flatulent colic, hiccup and diarrhoea due to indigestion. For treating these disorders, a drop of Dill oil, mixed in a teaspoon of honey sholud be licked immediately after meal. A drop of dill oil given with castor oil to young children prevents gripping pain in the abdomen and increases its purgative action by relaxing the intestines.

• Diarrhoea and dysentery

Dill possesses an anti-diarrhoeal activity. The seeds of this plant yield a very powerful carminative oil. These seeds, when roasted in ghee with fenugreek seeds in equal quantity, are a specific medicine for diarrhoea and acute bacillary dysentery. For better results, roasted seeds should be powdered and then mixed with curd or buttermilk for use in these conditions.

• Viral infections

Dill possesses antiviral property and helps fight infection. The seeds of this plant are especially effective in infections like colds and influenza. About 60 grams of infusion of the seeds, mixed with honey, should be given thrice daily in treating these disorders.

• Insomnia

The Dill is a calming and sedative food. It is an ancient remedy for insomnia. The Greeks used to put leaves of this plant in their cap or used to cover their heads with leaves to induce sleep. The Hindu physicians in ancient India also knew that keeping few springs of dill leaves near the pillow, while going to bed induces one to sleep soundly. In fact, the Hindi name of the plant is derived from the word 'sooya' which means slept.

• Pregnancy and lactation

Dill leaves are of great value to pregnant women and nursing mothers. Their liberal use after child birth increases breast milk. They also prevent early ovulation. Their regular use thus acts as a natural birth control device.

• Menstrual disorders

Dill is useful in stimulating and regulating menstrual flow. It is effective in spasmodic menstrual pain in young girls and absence of menstruation due to anaemia, exposure to cold and pregnancy. About 60 grams of decoction of the fresh leaves, mixed with a teaspoon of parsley juice, should be given thrice daily in the treatment of these disorders.

• Boils and swellings

A paste made from the fresh dill leaves can be applied as a

poultice to ripen blood boils. Its application with little turmeric powder prevents formation of pus in ulcers and heals them quickly. The leaves boiled in sesame oil make an excellent liniment for reducing swelling and pain of the joints.

Uses

The green plant is used fresh as a flavouring for soups, sauces and other culinary purposes. The seeds are used as a substitute for caraway seeds, as a flavouring in curry powder and medicinally as a source of dill-water, specially useful for flatulence in babies. The leaves can be added to vegetable salads. Leaves and seeds both can be used when making pickles or chutneys and cool summer drinks. This culinary herb is also a natural preservative, and in the days before refrigeration, vegetables were often pickled in vinegar or brine to preserve them. With dill added, they lasted even longer. Dill owes its preservative action to its ability to inhibit the growth of several bacteria.

Precautions

In sensitive persons, ingesting dill might cause skin rash, but the leaves, seeds and seed oil are generally considered non-toxic. If any skin irritation develops, its use should be discontinued.

It would be advisable for the expectant mothers to use this spice in small quantities daily as its excessive use may cause abortion.

Fennel

An Aid to Digestion

15

Description

The fennel *(Foenniculum)* is a yellowish green, biennial or perennial herb commonly cultivated throughout India. It has been used for flavouring from times immemorial. All parts of the plant are aromatic.

The Fennel is similar in appearance and flavour to Dill, although fennel has a more distinct, almost aniseed flavour. The two spices are also similar in that, both were noted as medicines in the records of Ancient Egypt. Fennel is often mistaken for aniseed as the flavour of the leaves and fruit resemble that of anise. However, fennel seed is not as strongly aromatic as aniseed, and is larger and pale lime-green in colour.

Origin and distribution

Fennel is a native of the Mediterranean region, where it has been cultivated since ancient times. It has become naturalized in many temperate countries and can be grown in the tropics. It is now widely cultivated in Bulgaria, Romania, Hungary, Greece, Turkey, Italy, France, Germany, Egypt, India, and China.

In Greek mythology, Prometheus concealed the fire of the sun in a hollow fennel stalk and brought it down to earth from Heaven for the human race. Pliny, an eminent Greek Physician declares that the herb enables the eye to perceive with clarity the beauty of nature. In ancient times, fennel juice was used as an effective cure in eye disorders like defective vision, night-blindness and cataract. It was an old custom to wash the eyes of a newborn baby with fennel water.

Nutritive value/Composition

An analysis of the fennel shows it to consist of moisture 6.30 percent, protein 9.5 percent, fat 10 percent, minerals 13.4 percent, fibre 18.5 percent and carbohydrates 42.3 percent per 100 grams. Its mineral and vitamin contents are calcium 1.3 mg.percent, phosphorus 0.48 mg. percent, iron 0.01 mg. percent, sodium 0.09 mg. percent, potassium 1.7 mg. percent, thiamine 9.41 mg. percent, riboflavin 0.36 mg. percent, niacin 600 mg, percent and vitamin C12 mg, percent. Its calorific value is 370.

The composition of the fennel oil varies widely, according to the variety or race from which the oil has been distilled and according to the region of origin. Indian fennel oil contains over 70 percent anethole and 6 percent fenchone. It possesses a sweet taste. Oils of good quality contain 50-70 percent anethole. The fatty acids of the oil are palmitic 4 mg. percent and petroselinic acid 60 mg. percent

Medicinal virtues

The leaves of fennel are digestive, appetizing and stimulant. They increase the secretion and discharge of urine. The seeds are sweet, laxative and aphrodisiac. They arrest secretion or bleeding, relieve flatulence and promote

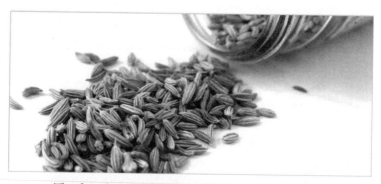

The fennel seeds are sweet, laxative and aphrodisiac.

the removal of catarrhal matter and phlegm from the bronchial tubes. Oil of fennel, distilled from the dry seeds is aromatic, carminative and antispasmodic. It is used in various carminative preparations. In Germany, fennel seed is licensed as a standard medicinal tea for dyspepsia. It is also used in cough syrups and honey, and stomach and bowel remedies, especially in pediatrics, as aqueous infusion. It is often used in combination with aniseed.

• Digestive Disorders

The use of fennel has been found beneficial in the treatment of digestive disorders. They are valuable food for relieving gas and expelling wind from the stomach. An infusion is prepared by boiling a tablespoon of fennel seeds in 100 ml of water for half an hour. This infusion is highly beneficial in the treatment of indigestion, biliousness and flatulence. Chewing its seeds everyday after meals prevents foul breath, indigestion, constipation and vomiting.

Fennel seeds may be given in small quantities to help young children to digest carbohydrates. A weak solution of fennel tea may be given to an uncomfortable baby, with or without milk, to help bring up wind and to soothe the baby.

• Colic

Fennel seeds are an effective remedy for colic. Their use can help the babies in the release of gas from the tummy. For better results they can be used in combination with other herbs like peppermint and crushed caraway seeds or alone. A teaspoon of the fennel seeds is boiled in a cup of water, and allowed to soak in the water for about 20 minutes. This is strained and allowed to cool. This tea, given to the baby in his feed bottle helps cure colic. Not more than a teaspoon or two should be given at a time.

• Respiratory disorders

The leaves and seeds of Fennel possess mucus clearing properties. They promote the removal of catarrhal matter and phlegm from the bronchial tubes. They are thus beneficial in the treatment of respiratory disorders like asthma and bronchitis. The juice of the leaves may be given for treating these diseases. Eating fennel seeds with figs is also a good medicine for cough, bronchitis and lung abscesses.

• Menstrual disorders

Fennel seeds promote menstruation and regulate monthly periods. An infusion of the seeds can be given in painful menstruation and other menstrual irregularities.

• Food Poisoning

Fennel roots and leaves are an antidote for food poisoning. They should be used in the form of tea.

• Eye Disorders

It is believed that fennel benefits the eyes. Herbalists today recommend bathing the weakened, sore or inflamed eye with fennel tea. Regular application of the leaf-juice, boiled with honey, is said to cure conjunctivitis and weakness of the eye.

• As beauty aid

Fennel can be used beneficially as a beauty aid. A strong, short brew of fennel may be prepared, cooled and then mixed with a teacup of yoghurt and a little honey. This mixture may be applied as a face pack. It will rejuvenate the skin.

Uses

The leaves are eaten raw in salads. Swollen stem bases are either used in salads or as a cooked vegetable. The fruits are used as a flavouring in soups, meat dishes and sauces. They are official in pharmacopoeias of many countries, because of the presence of a volatile oil. The oil is used in perfumes, soups and medicines.

Fenugreek

For Clean and Healthy Body

16

Description

Fenugreek *(Trigonella foenum graecum)* is an erect, legume, strongly scented, robust, annual plant, about 30 to 60 cm high. It has compound, smooth and thin leaves of light green colour, axillary yellow flowers and thin pointed pods 10 to 15 cm. long. Each pod contains 10 to 20 seeds, which are smooth and oblong, about 3mm long. They emit a peculiar odour and have flavour of their own. They are used as a spice.

Origin and distribution

Fenugreek is considered to be a native of south-Eastern Europe and West Asia. It is also found growing widely in North-western India. It has been used since ancient times both as a food and medicine by the people living on the shores of the Mediterranean and in Asia. It is extensively cultivated throughout Africa, India and Central and South America.

Nutritive value/Composition

An analysis of fenugreek seeds shows them to contain moisture 13.7 percent, protein 26.2 percent, fat 5.8 percent, minerals 3.0 percent, fibre 7.2 percent and carbohydrates 44.1 percent per 100 grams. Their mineral and vitamin contents are calcium 160 mg. percent, phosphorus 370 mg. percent, iron 14.1 mg. percent, carotene 96 meg. percent, thiamine 0.34 mg. percent, riboflavin 0.29 mg. percent and niacin 1.1 mg. percent per 100 grams. Their calorific value is 333.

The seeds of fenugreek contain six percent of a foetid, bitter fatty oil, 28 percent resin and mucilage and 22 percent albumin. The seeds contain alkaloid trigonelline, which the authoritative U.S. pharmacopeia describes as the methylbetaine of nicotinic acid — the pellagra preventive factor. They also contain choline, essential oil, saponin, volatile oil, bitter extractive and a yellow colouring substance. The seeds are rich in essential amino acids.

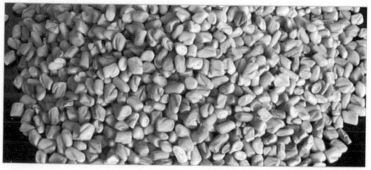

Fenugreek seeds are highly mucus-solvent and soothing agents.

Medicinal virtues

The seeds of the plant are the best cleansers within the body, highly mucus-solvents and soothing agents. They have antibiotic powers and they help control blood sugar in diabetes. The seeds are also antidiarrhoel, anti-ulcer and anticancer foods. They tend to lower blood pressure and help prevent intestinal gas.

• Digestive Disorders

Fenugreek seeds are useful in digestive system disorders like colic, flatulence, dysentery and dyspepsia. To treat flatulence, a teaspoon of the seeds should be soaked overnight in a cup of water. The next morning, the water should be drunk and seeds eaten.

• Diarrhoea

The seeds of fenugreek are a powerful anti-diarrhoeal food. Their use has been found effective in controlling diarrhoea. Half a teaspoon of these seeds should be taken with water three times daily. They have long been used as a folk remedy for diarrhoea in India and Middle East. According to Dr. Krishna C. Srivastava at Odense University in Denmark, this remedy produces quick and marked relief usually after the second dose.

• Anaemia

The seeds of fenugreek are valuable in anaemia, being rich in iron. They should be taken in the same manner as for flatulance.

• Fever

A tea made from fenugreek seeds is equal in value to quinine for reducing fevers. It is particularly valuable as a cleansing and soothing drink. The fenugreek seeds, when moistened with water are themselves slightly mucilaginous. A tea made from them has power to dissolve more sticky substance as body mucus.

• Stomach disorders

This tea soothes inflamed stomach and intestines and cleanses the stomach, bowels, kidneys and respiratory tract of excess mucus. It is beneficial in the healing of peptic ulcers as the mild coating of mucilaginous material deposited by fenugreek, as it passes through the stomach and intestines, provides a protective shell for the ulcers. For treating ulcers, a teaspoon of the seeds should be taken in the morning on an empty stomach, and then a cup of chilled milk with two crushed cardamom should be drunk. This treatment should be continued for 7 to 15 days.

• Respiratory infections

During the early acute stages of any of the respiratory tract infections, such as bronchitis, influenza, sinusitis, catarrh and suspected pneumonia, fenugreek tea will help the body to produce perspiration, dispel toxicity and shorten the period of fever. Four cups of this tea should be taken daily and the quantity reduced as condition improves.

• Sore throat

A gargle made from fenugreek seeds is the best for ordinary sore throat. When preparing a gargle, the solution should be much stronger than a tea. Two tablespoons of fenugreek seeds should be put into a litre of cold water and allowed to simmer for half an hour over a low flame. It should be allowed to cool to a bearable temperature, strained and entire quantity is then used as a gargle.

• Diabetes

Fenugreek seeds have been found highly effective in the treatment of diabetes. According to research studies conducted at National Institute of Nutrition, Hyderabad, fenugreek seeds, when given in varying doses of 25 grams to 100 grams daily, diminish reactive hyperglycemia in diabetic patients. Levels of glucose, serum cholesterol and tryglycerides were also significantly reduced in the diabetes patients when the seeds were consumed. These studies indicate that the effect of taking fenugreek seeds could be quite dramatic, when consumed with 1200-1400 calories diet per day, which is usually recommended for diabetic patients.

Fenugreek seeds can be consumed by diabetics in different ways. A teaspoon of the seeds can be swallowed with water daily. In the alternative, the seeds can be soaked overnight in water and can be taken first thing in the morning. The soaked seeds can also be dried and powdered and this powder is taken with milk in doses of one teaspoon twice daily.

• High blood cholesterol

Fenugreek seeds are considered a cholesterol lowering food. Daniel Mowrey of the American Phytotherapy Research Laboratory in Salt Lake City, Utah, firmly believes that they reduce cholesterol. Israeli scientists at Hebrew University of Jerusalem have shown that fenugreek seeds can lower blood sugar and cholesterol in both diabetics and healthy people. Additionally, they have identified an active ingredient in fenugreek seeds. It is a gel-like soluble fibre called galactomannan. In animal studies, the fenugreek gel binds up bile acids, lowering cholesterol, much the same way as common drugs do.

• Sexual weakness

Since ancient times fenugreek has been held in high esteem as a tonic for the reproductive system. Pliny, the ancient Roman sage, who wrote a lengthy discourse on spice remedies and quoted many herbal and medical authorities, says that fenugreek has a beneficial effect on the sex organ. To this day, the Turkish maidens of Tunisia still prepare and eat a mixture of honey and powdered fenugreek seed to improve their feminine figures and sexy appearance.

The oil contained in fenugreek seed could account for the plant's ancient reputation as a sex rejuvenator for the person deficient in vitamin A and D. For the last several years the damaging effects on the male organs resulting from vitamin A deficiency in the diet has been under scientific study.

Another possible sex-rejuvenating property contained in fenugreek is trimethylamine. Scientific studies show that it acts as a sex hormone in frogs, enabling them to prepare for mating.

• Menstrual and menopausal disorders

In American folk medicine, fenugreek was considered a potent menstruation promoter. It became a key ingredient in Lydia E. Pinkham's Vegetable compound, one of the 19th-century America's most popular patent medicines for 'female weakness". Almost a century after Lydia Pinkham's death, scientists have confirmed that fenugreek seeds contain chemicals similar to the female sex hormone estrogen. Loss of estrogen causes menopausal symptoms, so adding fenugreek to the diet might minimize them.

• Pregnancy and Lactation

The seeds are fried in ghee and finely powdered. This powder is mixed with wheat flour and sugar to prepare a halwa. This preparation, taken in small quantity daily, helps in quick normalization after delivery. The seeds, made into a gruel, are given as diet to nursing mothers for increasing the flow of milk.

• Deadened sense

The seeds help restore a deadened sense of taste or smell. The loss of sense of taste occurs due to improper functioning of the salivary glands. They often become plugged with mucus and accumulated juices, causing swelling. Similarly, the sense of smell is obstructed due to long accumulations of mucus or other impurities in the nose where the olfactory nerves are based. Regular use of fenugreek has proved beneficial in both these cases.

• Dandruff

Fenugreek seeds are useful in the removal of dandruff. Two tablespoons of the seeds should be soaked overnight in water. In the morning, the softened seeds should be ground into a fine paste. This paste should be applied all over the scalp and left on the head for half an hour. The hair should then be washed thoroughly with soapnut solution or *shikakai*. Paste of the fresh leaves of fenugreek applied over the scalp regularly is also useful in dandruff.

• Leucorrhoea

Fenugreek, taken both internally as a tea and used as a douche, is very effective in reliving leucorrhoea which plagues a good majority of civilised women and which only denotes a cattarnal condition of the female organs. For a douche, the solution can be prepared in the same manner as for a throat gargle.

• Bad breath and body odour

The tea made from fenugreek seeds is also beneficial in the case of bad breath and body odour. Unpleasant odours emanate from body openings due to accumulations of hardened mucus and other poisons in the nasal and oral passages, the gastrointestinal tract, the urinary tract, the bloodstream and vagina. Fenugreek tea, taken regularly will help remove these accumulations from such spots where mouth wash and soap can never penetrate.

• As beauty aid

Paste of the fresh leaves applied over the scalp regularly, before taking bath, lengthens hair, preserves the natural colour and keeps the hair silky soft. This paste, applied on the face every night before going to bed and washed with warm water, prevents pimples, blackheads, dryness of the face and early appearance of wrinkles. It improves complexion and makes one look years younger.

Uses

Fresh tender pods, leaves and shoots are eaten as cooked vegetable since ancient times in India, Egypt and other countries. In Indian homes, seeds are generally used as a condiment and for flavouring. They form an ingredient of curry powder. They are also used in bread and bakery products.

17

Garlic

An All-Round Wonder Drug

Description

The garlic *(Allium sativum)*, a condiment crop of the onion family, has been cultivated from time immemorial. It has been variously described as a food, a herb, a medicinal plant and an antidote to evil by various people at different times throughout the ages. It has long been recognised all over the world as an all-round wonder drug for the treatment of several diseases.

Garlic is an erect, hardy, bulbous perennial plant, normally grown annually. The plant is smooth and shiny, and grows upto 30 cm. in height. It has irregular roots, condensed, flattened stem and narrow flat leaves. It bears small white flowers and bulb. The bulb consists six to 35 bulblets called cloves which are enclosed in a thin whitish, glistering and transparent covering. Garlic has a stronger flavour than onion.

Origin and distribution

Garlic is believed to have originated in Central Asia and was known to the Chinese as far back as 3,000 B.C. It continues to be one of the staple item of China's diet even today. It was distributed at an early date to Mediterranean region. Garlic was being grown in ancient China, Egypt, Greece and Rome and was used both as a staple food and a medicine for several ailments. It spread to all parts of the world and is now widely grown in the Mediterranean area, India, the Philippines, China, Ethiopia, Kenya, Brazil and Mexico. In India, it has long been cultivated practically in all parts of the country as an important condiment crop.

Nutritive values/Composition

An analysis of garlic shows it to contain moisture 62.0 percent, protein 6.3 percent, fat 0.1 percent, minerals 1.0 percent, fibre 0.8 percent and carbohydrates 29.8 percent per 100 grams of edible portion. Its mineral and vitamin contents are calcium 30 mg. percent, phosphorus 310 mg. percent, iron 1.3 mg. percent, thiamine 0.06 mg. percent, riboflavin 0.23 mg. percent, niacin 0.4 mg. percent and vitamin C 13 mg. percent. It also contains traces of iodine, sulphur and chlorine. Its calorific value is 145.

The bulbs yield an essential oil containing allyl propyl disulphide, diallyl disulphide and two other sulphur compounds. They also contain antiseptic and hypotensive, or causing low blood pressure pinciples-allicin, allisatin I and allisatin II.

Medicinal virtues

Garlic has been held in high esteem for its health-building qualities for centuries all over the world. Khnoum Khoufouf, the builder of one of the oldest pyramids, (4500 B.C.) was among the first to recognise the true virtues of garlic, for he decreed that all his workers should take garlic every day so that they could maintain their health and strength.

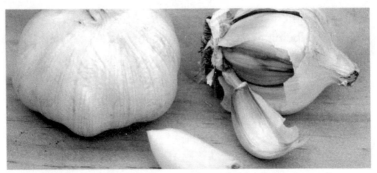

Garlic lowers blood pressure and blood cholesterol,
prevents blood clots, heart attacks and cancer.

Garlic has been used to treat an array of ills since the dawn of civilization. It is a proven broad-spectrum antibiotic that combats bacteria, intestinal parasites and viruses. Garlic lowers blood pressure and blood cholesterol, discourages dangerous blood clotting and helps prevent cancer and heart attacks. It acts as a decongestant, expectorant, antispasmodic and anti-inflammatory agent. It boosts immune system, relieves gas and possesses antidiarrhoel, oestrogenic and diuretic properties.

• Infectious diseases

Garlic is one of nature's strongest, anti-bacterial foods due to Allicin contained in it. One milligram of this substance equals to 15 Oxford units of penicillin. Tests show that garlic kills or cripples at least 72 infectious bacteria that spread diarrhoea, dysentery, tuberculosis and encephalitis, among other diseases.

Infections like cholera, typhoid and dysentery caused by organisms can readily become resistant to antibiotic therapy. They are all life threatening and are still endemic in many countries today. Garlic is one of the most effective remedies for these disorders. Its action has been confirmed against the specific classes of bacteria responsible for these diseases in laboratory test.

According to Dr. F.W. Crosman an eminent physician, garlic is a marvelous remedy for pneumonia, if given in sufficient quantities. Thus physicians used garlic for many years in pneumonia, and said that in no instance did it fail to bring down the temperature as well as the pulse and respiration, within 48 hours. Garlic juice can also be applied externally to the chest with beneficial results, as it is an irritant and rubefacient.

Garlic is considered an excellent remedy for diphtheria. Chewing a clove of garlic removes the membranes, reduces temperature and relieves the patient. About 30 to 60 gms of garlic can be used in this way in three or four hours. For a week after the membrane disappears, 30 to 60 gms of garlic should be chewed daily. The diphtheric patient has no taste or smell and merely finds the garlic hot.

Garlic works as an antibiotic in various forms. Raw garlic taken orally kills infectious bacteria in the intestines directly. Crushed garlic in water is used as a douche or a clove of garlic inserted in vagina kills infectious organisms in the vaginal tract. Garlic nose drops directly kill the viruses, which cause cold or influenza. Bacteria and viruses in the lungs and bronchial tract can be killed by Garlic's sulphur compounds, absorbed either through food, or inhalation or poultices, and then excreted through the lungs.

Infusion of the garlic is an excellent antiseptic lotion. It can be successfully used in washing the foul-smelling chronic ulcers, cut wounds and carbuncles. Garlic juice with three parts of distilled water has been employed as a lotion for cleansing infected wounds. Definite improvement is noticed within 24 hours and substantial improvement within 48 hours. Application of dressing containing 15 percent garlic juice once a day over an ulcer removes pus in few days. It also relieves pain within a short time.

• Blood clots

Garlic is a powerful anti-coagulant food. It effectively prevents dangerous blood clotting. Even in moderate dietary amounts, it will help thin the blood, thereby reducing its tendency to form blood clots within the arteries. This was discovered by research scientist in the mid-70s. Studies were conducted in India on Jain religious sect. While some Jains abstain completely from onions and garlic, on religious grounds, others eat large amounts of them. A third group eats a moderate amount.

The three population groups are very similar in most other respect, making it easier for a controlled study of garlic and onion. Those Jains who eat garlic and onions liberally consumed nearly 500 grams of onions and at least 17 garlic cloves in a week. It was found that the blood of this people had less tendency to clot than the blood of the other groups, and the group that did not eat garlic and onion at all had the highest tendency to clot.

Drugs that thin blood are often prescribed after strokes, heart attacks, or blood clots in the legs or lungs. The use of Garlic can interfere and render this drug more potent and as well reduce the side effects from improper doses. Garlic does not appear to make much difference whether it is taken raw or in cooked form for its blood-thinning effects.

• Depression

The use of garlic helps elevate mood and is thus beneficial in the treatment of depression. Many researchers studying garlic for its effects on blood and cholesterol noticed that those who ate garlic experienced a definite lift in mood and had a greater feeling of well-being. This was especially noted by a German researcher at University of Hanover. He recently tested a special garlic preparation on people with high cholesterol. The garlic eater according to questionnaires felt much better after the garlic therapy. They experienced notably less fatigue, anxiety, sensitivity, agitation and irritability. The power of garlic as mood elevator can be attributed to its richness in selenium and its antioxidant activity.

• High blood pressure

Garlic is an ancient folk remedy to lower blood pressure. It has been used in China as a blood pressure lowering medication for a very long time and is now widely used in Germany for this purpose. It helps reduce blood pressure and tension because of its power to ease the spasm of the small arteries. Garlic also slows the pulse, modifies the heart rhythm, besides relieving the symptoms of dizziness, numbness, shortness of breath and the formation of gas within the digestive track. The average dosage should be two to three capsules a day to make a dent in the blood pressure.

In a German test of Kwai, doses of garlic preparation equivalent to a couple of daily garlic cloves reduced diastolic blood pressure in patients with mild high blood pressure. The blood pressure in the garlic group came down from an average 171/102 to 152/89 after three months, while the blood pressure of the placebo group remains the same. Interestingly, garlic's impact increased stronger throughout the test, suggesting that daily infusions of garlic have a cumulative effect. Both raw and cooked garlic can lower blood pressure, although raw garlic is thought to be more powerful.

• Asthma

Garlic is an excellent mucus clearing food. It is an effective expectorant and helps remove mucus from the bronchial tube. Allicin, which gives garlic its flavour, is converted in the body to a drug similar to S-carboxymethylcysteine (Mucodyne), a classic European lung medication that regulates mucus flow.

Egyptians and Romans in ancient times and Arabs and Persians in medieval times, all used garlic to treat asthma. Even conventional physicians in Germany and United States used it as a remedy for asthma in the first half of the twentieth century. The biochemical mechanism involved may be that garlic affects substances called prostaglandins in the body. To derive this benefit, garlic must be heated or cooked. An effective method to take garlic in asthma is to boil three cloves in 30 ml. of milk and take once daily. Steaming ginger tea with minced garlic cloves in it can also help to keep the problem under control and should be taken both in the morning and evening.

• Digestive system disorders

Garlic is one of the most valuable foods for the digestive system. It exercises a beneficial effect on the lymph, aids in elimination of noxious waste matter from the body. It stimulates peristaltic action and the secretion of the digestive juices. Crushed cloves of garlic may be infused in water or milk and taken for all disorders of the digestion. It has an antiseptic effect and is an excellent remedy for infectious diseases and inflammations of the stomach and intestine. The oil of garlic is absorbed into the alimentary tract and is eliminated partly through the urine.

Garlic produces a very marked effect on the intestine. It is an excellent agent as a worm expeller. It also has a soothing effect on the various forms of diarrhoea. Problems such as colitis, dysentery and many other intestinal upsets can be successfully treated with fresh garlic or garlic capsules. Garlic has the ability to destroy harmful bacteria in the intestines without affecting the beneficial organisms that aid digestion.

• Rheumatic afflictions

Garlic possesses anti-inflammatory property. It is known to affect prostaglandin that helps reduce inflammation. Physicians in India noticed during a study of garlic's impact on heart disease that garlic eaters often got relief from joint pain, in particular those with osteoarthritis, which also involves inflammation. During the test, subjects ate two or three raw or cooked garlic cloves every day.

In Russia, garlic is used extensively in the treatment of rheumatism and associated diseases. In Britain also, garlic is recommended to rheumatic sufferers. Experiments in Japan tested a garlic extract on patients with lumbago and arthritis and a large number benefited, without any undesirable side effects.

Garlic is also one of the most effective food medicines in sciatica. It can be used in the form of either raw garlic or garlic milk. In case of raw garlic, it should be cut into small pieces and taken with a teaspoon of honey with each meal. Garlic milk can be prepared both in cooked and uncooked states. Uncooked form is more powerful. This milk is prepared by adding the pulp of the crushed garlic in uncooked buffalo milk. The proportion is four cloves to 110 ml of milk. In cooked state, it should be boiled in milk. The most popular method is to take the garlic cloves internally, although some reports indicate that pain can also be relieved by rubbing the affected parts with cloves of cut garlic. Garlic oil is rapidly absorbed through the skin and into the bloodstream and quickly reaches the affected areas.

• High blood cholesterol

The use of garlic has been found highly beneficial in treatment of high blood cholesterol. About 20 published human tests show that fresh garlic and some garlic preparations reduce cholesterol substantially. According to Robert Lin, Ph.D., of the First World Conference on the health aspects of garlic, three fresh garlic cloves a day can lower cholesterol by 10 percent on an average and up to 15 percent in some cases. It does not matter whether the garlic is cooked or raw, he says. It is effective both ways. Six compounds in garlic have been identified that lower cholesterol by reducing liver's synthesis of cholesterol.

In a test, at L.T.M. Medical College in Mumbai, 50 persons ate three raw garlic cloves every morning for two months. Their cholesterol came down by 15 percent from an average 5.54 to 4.68. Their blood clotting factors also improved dramatically. In another study, at Bastyr College in Seattle, a daily dose of garlic oil from three fresh garlic cloves brought cholesterol down by seven percent in a month, but, more important, raised good-type HDL by 23 percent.

• Cancer

Garlic contains multiple anti-cancer compounds and antioxidant and tops the American National Cancer Institute's list as a potential cancer-preventive food. It lessens the chances of stomach cancer in particular. More than 30 different compounds have been isolated from garlic, which are potent enemies of carcinogens. These compounds include diallyl sulphide, quercetin and ajoene. In animals, they block the most terrifying cancer-causing agents such as nitrosamines and aflatoxin, linked specifically to stomach, lung and liver cancer. Feeding garlic to animals consistently blocks cancer.

Garlic may also interfere with the progress of cancer. A study found that garlic compounds are toxic to malignant cells. Thus, garlic substances might help destroy cancerous cells somewhat the way chemotherapy drugs do. In the German study of human cells, one potent garlic compound, ajoene, was three times as toxic to malignant cells as to normal cells.

Garlic might also discourage colon and stomach cancers by functioning as an antibiotic. New research studies suggest that an infection by H.pylori bacteria contributes to these cancers. If so, says Dr. Tim Byers of the Centers for Disease Control and Prevention; garlic might fight cancer by attacking the bacteria.

• Meningitis

Garlic has now been found to be effective in the treatment of the dreaded meningitis, most fatal disease-affecting children. A Chinese medical journal reported that of the 26 cases of meningitis treated with garlic by Chinese physicians, 16 were totally cured. In five other cases, all symptoms of the brain disease vanished within few days of treatment and the remaining five cases ended fatally.

• Fevers

Garlic can be used beneficially in the treatment of fevers. About 20 gms. of Garlic should be boiled in 1:1 cup mixture of milk and water till it is reduced to half the quantity. It should be taken either at bed-time or before breakfast. In case of typhoid fever, a teaspoon of Garlic juice should be given mixed in either jaggery syrup or fruit juice, every four hours.

• Whooping cough

Garlic is an excellent remedy for whooping cough. Syrup of garlic should be given in doses of five drops to a teaspoon

two or three times a day in treating this condition. It should
be given more often if the coughing is frequent and violent.

• Earache

The use of garlic has been found valuable in earache. Three
grams of garlic should be boiled well in 60 ml. of gingelly
(til) oil. It should be cooled and filtered. This can be used as
ear drops, two to three drops may *be* put in the ear in treating
this condition.

• Sexual impotence

Garlic is a natural, harmless and powerful aphrodisiac food.
Its regular use imparts sexual vigour and vitality. Dr.
Robinson, an eminent sexologist of America considers that
garlic has a pronounced aphrodisiac effect. It is a tonic for
loss of sexual power from any cause and for sexual debility
and impotency from over indulgence in sex and nervous
exhaustion from dissipating habit. Its use has been found
especially valuable for elder persons of high nervous tension
and failing sexual power.

• Strengthens immune system

Garlic greatly helps stimulate immune functioning. Its antibacterial, anti-viral and anti-cancer activities are partly due to
its ability to enhance immune functioning. It particularly
stimulates the power of T-lymphocytes and macrophages,
which play a dominant role in immune functions. This has
been discovered by Benjamin H.S. Lau, M.D., of the school
of Medicine at Loma Linda University. In laboratory tests, he
found that garlic extract impeled macrophages to generate
more agents to kill microbes and tumour cells. Dr. Lau calls
garlic a biological response modifier.

Several years ago, Dr. Tariq Abdullah, M.D., and colleague at the Akbar Clinic and Research Center in Panama City, Florida, ate large amounts of raw garlic, up to 15 cloves a day. Others in the study ate no garlic. The blood from the garlic eaters had more natural killer cells. In fact, such natural killer cells, destroyed from 140-160 percent more cells than did natural killer cells derived from non-garlic eaters. An amount as small as 1.8 grams of garlic, about half a clove, results in an increase in natural killer cell activity.

Uses

In India, garlic is used for centuries in the preparation of curries, various chutneys, pickles, vegetables with gravies and tomato ketchup.

Precaution

Excessive use of garlic should be avoided. High doses of raw garlic — more than three cloves a day — can cause gas, bloating, diarrhoea and fever in some persons. Excessive use of garlic can also cause heat in the body and burning sensation during urination. Garlic's strong-smelling compounds are often eliminated through skin and lungs. Fresh parsley may be chewed to eliminate the odour in the breath. During pregnancy and lactation, excessive garlic intake might cause heartburn. It may also affect the taste of mother's milk.

Ginger

A Great Food Medicine

18

Description

Ginger *(Zingiber officinale)* is one of the most important spices of India. It has been used in Asia since ancient times and is one of the earliest oriental spices known to Europe. It contributes greatly towards health and is regarded as a medicine for several ailments.

Ginger is a large tuberous horizontal perennial plant having knots. It grows upto a height of 90 cm. It has underground branching stems *(rhizomes)* which are swollen and tough. They are white or yellow outside and become grey-brown or orange with age, upto 2.5 cm. in diameter. The leaves are 15-30 cm. long, 2-3 cm. broad. The leaves and rhizomes have characteristic fragrant odour when cut or bruised. Rhizomes are dug out after the leafy parts are dried. They are sold as fresh ginger in the market or are peeled, sliced and dried. The dried ginger is known as *sount* in vernacular.

Origin and distribution

Ginger is believed to have originated in India and was introduced in China at a very early date. It appears to have been used as a spice and a medicine from early times by the Indians and Chinese. There are numerous references to ginger in Sanskrit literature and in Chinese Medical treatises. It was known in Europe in first century A.D. and was mentioned by Dioscorides and Pliny. It was brought by Arab traders from India. The Sanskrit name *Singabera* gave rise to the Greek *Zingiberi* and to the late latin *Zingiberi*.

The Arabs took the plant from India to East Africa in the 13th century and the Portuguese to West Africa and other parts of the tropics in the 16th century. As living rhizomes of ginger are very easy to transport, the plant soon spread to all tropical countries. It is now cultivated extensively in almost all tropical and subtropical countries, especially China, India, Nigeria, Australia, Jamaica, and Haiti. China and India are the world's leading producers of ginger. It is cultivated all over India, but ginger grown in Kerala is found to be superior than other places in aroma and in taste.

Nutritive value/Composition

An analysis of the fresh ginger shows it to contain moisture 80.9 percent, protein 2.3 percent, fat 0.9 percent, minerals 1.2 percent, fibre 2.4 percent and carbohydrates 12.3 percent per 100 grams. Its mineral and vitamin contents are calcium 20 mg. percent, phosphorus 60 mg. percent, iron 2.6 mg. percent, carotene 40 meg. percent, thiamine 0.06 mg. percent and vitamin C 6 mg. percent per 100 grams. Its calorific value is 67.

The composition of ginger varies with type or variety, region, agro-climatic conditions, methods of curing, dying, packaging and storage. Chemical analysis of 26 varieties of ginger grown in India was conducted at CFTRI, Mysore, which showed the following range of important qualities: volatile oil 1.0 to 2.7 percent, oleoresin (acetone extract) 3.9 to 9.3 percent, water extract 14.4 to

25.8 percent, cold alcohol extract 3.5 to 9.3 percent, starch 40.4 to 59.0 percent, total ash 5.1 to 9.3 percent, water soluble ash 3.9 to 8.84 percent, acid insoluble ash 0.0 to 0.59 percent and alkalinity of ash 25.7 to 79.0 ml. of 0.1 N HCl per 100 gm. of unpeeled ginger.

On steamed distillation, dried, cracked and comminuted ginger yields 1.0 to 3.0 percent of pale yellow, viscid oil. This oil possesses the aromatic odour but not the pungent flavour of the spice.

Medicinal virtues

Ginger is being used in India from Vedic period and is called *Maha-Aushadi,* meaning the great medicine. It has been used for centuries in Asia to treat a variety of diseases like nausea, vomiting, headache, chest congestion, cholera, colds, diarrhoea, stomachache, rheumatism and nervous diseases.

Today, ginger is official in the national pharmacopeias of Austria, China, Egypt, Germany, Great Britain, Japan, and Switzerland. The *British Herbal Compendium* indicates ginger for atonic dyspepsia, colic, prophylaxis of travel sickness, and vomiting during pregnancy. It is also used for anorexia, bronchitis and rheumatic complaints. It is a

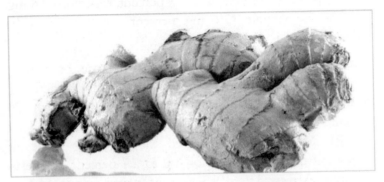

Ginger ranks high in antioxidant and anticancer activity.

powerful antioxidant. It also ranks very high in anticancer activity.

• Digestive system disorders

Ginger is a valuable drug for disorders of the digestive system. It is extremely useful in dyspepsia, flatulence, colic, nausea, vomiting, spasms and other painful affections of the stomach and the bowels, unattended by fever. Chewing a fresh piece of ginger after meals regularly is an insurance against these ailments. This protective action is attributable to excessive secretion of saliva, diastase enzyme and volatile oil.

Chewing a small 2.5 cm long piece of ginger with little salt before meals, improves the appetite and taste and cleanses the tongue and throat. Half a teaspoon of fresh ginger juice, mixed with one teaspoon of fresh lime juice and fresh mint juice and a tablespoon of honey, is an effective medicine for dyspepsia, nausea and vomiting due to bilousness, indigestion caused by intake of heavy non-vegetarian and fried fatty food, morning sickness, jaundice and piles. This mixture must be sucked thrice daily in the treatment of these conditions.

Dry or fresh ginger is highly beneficial in diarrhoea caused by indigestion. A piece of dry ginger should be powdered along with a crystal of rock salt, and a quarter teaspoon of this powder should be taken with a small piece of jaggery. It will bring quick relief as ginger, being carminative, aids digestion by stimulating the gastrointestinal track.

• Infectious diseases

Ginger is an antibiotic and helps fight infection. It has been used for centuries to treat many infectious diseases like cholera, diarrhoea and chest congestion. Its use has been found especially effective in whooping cough. A teaspoon of fresh ginger juice, mixed with a cup of fenugreek decoction and honey to taste, acts as an expectorant and diaphoretic in treating this disease. The fenugreek decoction can be made by boiling one teaspoon of seeds in 250 ml of water till it is reduced to half. The decoction of fenugreek is prepared by mixing one tablespoon of fenugreek seeds in a cupful of water. This mixture of ginger juice and fenugreek decoction should be taken both in the morning and evening.

• Rheumatic afflictions

Ginger is a powerful anti-inflammatory drug. It has been used for centuries in Ayurvedic system of medicine to treat various rheumatic and musculoskeletal diseases. In a recent study, Dr. Krishna C. Srivastava of Odense University in Denmark, tested ginger in small doses daily on a group of arthritis patients for three months. Most of them had less pain, swelling and morning stiffness and more mobility. Dr. Srivastava, who has successfully treated several arthritis patients with ginger, recommends an intake of 5 grams of fresh ginger or half a gram ground ginger three times a day. The ground ginger should be taken after dissolving in liquid. The experts opine that ginger seems to have no side effects.

Ginger presumably works in two or even more ways. It blocks formation of both prostaglandins and other inflammatory substances called leukotrienes. Further, Dr. Srivastava suggests that ginger's antioxidant activity breaks down inflammatory acids in the joints' synovial fluid. Dr. Srivastava has also found powdered dry ginger effective in combating pain and swelling from the inflammation of osteoarthritis.

• Blood clots

Blood can be kept free of dangerous clots by eating liberal quantities of ginger. This was discovered by Dr. Charles R.

Dorso, M.D. of Cornell University Medical College. He ate large quantity of Crabtree & Evelyn Ginger with Grapefruit Marmalade which was 15 percent ginger. When his blood did not coagulate as usual, he did a test by mixing some ground ginger with his own blood platelets, and found them to be less sticky. According to Dr. Dorso the active agent in ginger is gingerol which chemically resembles aspirin.

Ginger clamps down on the production of thromboxane, which is a potent promoter of platelet clumping. According to Dr. Krishna C Srivastava of Odense University in Denmark, ginger compounds are strong inhibitors of prostaglandin synthesis than the drug indomethacin, known for its potency.

• Viral diseases

Ginger possesses anti-viral activity. It destroys influenza viruses. A teaspoon of fresh ginger juice mixed with a cup of fenugreek decoction and honey to taste is an excellent diaphoretic mixture to reduce fever in influenza.

Ginger is an excellent remedy for coughs and colds. Extracted juice of ginger with honey should be taken three or four times a day in case of coughs. In case of colds, ginger should be cut into small pieces and boiled in a cup of water. It should then be strained and some jaggery or honey added to it. It should be drunk while hot. For chronic cold, a tea can be prepared by boiling half a teaspoon each of ginger paste, cloves and cinnamon powder. This should be drunk after adding a little honey to it.

• Respiratory disorders

Ginger is an expectorant food. It helps clear phlegm from the bronchial tube and is thus valuable in asthma, bronchitis, tuberculosis of the lungs and catarrh. A teaspoon of fresh ginger juice, mixed with a cup of fenugreek decoction and honey to taste, is an excellent medicine in treatment of these conditions.

A specific remedy for treating bronchitis is a mixture of half a teaspoon each of ginger powder, pepper and cloves. This mixture should be taken thrice daily. It may be licked with honey or taken as an infusion.

For treating Catarrah a piece each of ginger and turmeric should be ground together. Lime juice and some mustard oil should be added to three fourth of this mixture. This preparation may be applied all over the body, especially on the face, armpits, ears and neck. Warm water bath should be taken after half an hour and thereafter, the remaining one fourth of the mixture should be eaten with jaggery. This treatment should be taken for three days in the first week, for two days in the second week and one day in the third week.

• Aches and pains

Ginger is an excellent painkiller. It can cure all types of pain. In headache, ginger ointment made by rubing dry ginger with a little water and applied to the forehead offers relief. Backache can also be relieved by applying Ginger paste on the affected area. It allays toothache, burnt ginger mixed with common salt is rubbed over the teeth to cure dental sensitiveness caused by eating sour fruits. In case of earache, a few drops of ginger juice will give relief.

• Sexual debility

Ginger juice is a valuable aphrodisiac. It is highly beneficial in the treatment of sexual weakness. For better results, half a teaspoon of ginger juice should be taken with half-boiled egg and honey once daily at night for a month. It tones up the sex centers and cures impotency, premature ejaculation and spermatorrhoea.

• Menstrual disorders

Ginger is useful in menstrual disorders like painful menstruation and absence or stoppage of the menstrual flow due to exposure to cold winds and taking cold bath. A piece of fresh ginger should be pounded and boiled in a cup of water for few minutes. This infusion, should be taken with honey thrice daily after meals as a medicine in treating these conditions. Another method of taking ginger in case of painful menstruation is to mix one teaspoon each of the juices of Margosa leaves and ginger, and take two teaspoons of the mixed juice once daily for three to five days from the first day of menstruation.

• Migraine

The use of ginger is considered highly beneficial in the prevention and treatment of migraine. According to Dr. Krishna C Srivastava, ginger, like aspirin and some other sophisticated antimigraine drugs, affects prostaglandins, the body's hormone like substances that help control inflammatory responses involving histamine and pain. Ginger acts much like aspirin in blocking prostaglandin synthesis, leading to reduction in inflammation and pain.

• Dropsy

Ginger is also valuable in dropsy associated with scanty urination. A teaspoon of ginger juice mixed with a glass of tender coconut water makes an effective medicine for treating this condition.

• Boils

The use of ginger as an external application has been found beneficial in the treatment of boils. A paste of ginger powder mixed with equal quantity of turmeric powder can be applied on boils with beneficial results.

Uses

Ginger is available in two forms, fresh and dried. Both the forms are effective. Usually fresh ginger is used in the culinary preparations to increase aroma, taste and appetite. As the taste of ginger is not very good, it is mostly used in cooked vegetables. It is a common constituent of curry powder.

19

Liquorice
A Rejuvenating Spice

Description

Liquorice *(Glycyrrhiza glabra)* is a popular flavouring agent. It is a tall perennial plant, upto about 1.5 m. high. It has wrinkled woody root stock which is brown on the outside and yellow on the inside. The stem is round on the lower part and angular higher up. The leaves are egg-shaped and dark-green in colour. The flowers are yellow, purple or violet. Fruits are 1 to 3 cm. long, flat and densely covered all over with small spinous outgrowths. The dried roots and underground stems of the plant constitute the drug.

Origin and distribution

Liquorice grows wild and is cultivated in southern Europe, Syria, Iraq, Turkey, Greece and Russia. In India, it is cultivated in Jammu and Kashmir, Punjab and the sub-Himalayan region. The plant is found growing in the North-West provinces in Pakistan in a wild state.

Nutritive value/Composition

The chief constituent of liquorice is glycyrrhizin, which is present in the drug in the form of potassium and calcium salts of glycyrrhizic acid. Glycyrrhiza acid is not a glycoside since it yields on hydrolysis, one molecule of glycyrrhetic acid and two molecules of glycuronic acid but no sugar. Liquorice also contains glucose upto 3.8 percent, sucrose 2.4 to 6.5 percent, bitter principles, resins, mannite, asparagine 2 to 4 percent, and fat 0.8 percent.

Medicinal virtues

Liquorice has been known in pharmacy for thousands of years. In old Chinese pharmacy, it was considered to be a first class drug and rejuvenating property was ascribed to it, especially when used for long periods. It was used to allay thirst, feverishness, pain, cough and distress breathing. For many centuries China has used large quantities of liquorice and its many preparations are still sold there.

Liquorice is a potent, multi-faceted medicine. It has strong anticancer powers, possibly because of a high concentration of glycyrrhizin. Mice drinking glycyrrhizin dissolved in water have fewer skin cancers. It also kills bacteria, fights ulcers and diarrhoea. It may act as a diuretic.

Liquorice plays an important part in Hindu medicine and is one of the principal drugs of the 'Susruta'. It was also

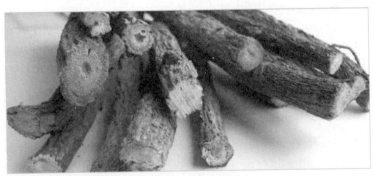

Liquorice is a multi-faceted medicine with strong anti-cancer powers.

frequently used in ancient Egypt, Greece and Rome. The root of the plant is laxative and expectorant. It has a soothing effect on the skin. The powdered liquorice is very popular in western medicine.

• Stomach distress

Liquorice is an excellent remedy for relieving pain, discomfort and other symptoms caused by acid matter in the stomach. Liquorice, when used in powder form helps to remove irritating effects of acid in a better way than alkalis. Roots of Liquorice boiled in water and then steamed can also relieve stomach upset. A teaspoon of this decoction should be mixed with equal quantity of honey and taken thrice daily.

• Peptic ulcer

Liquorice possesses anti ulcer activity. According to Dr. James Duke, Ph.D. and Botanist at the U.S. Department of Agriculture, liquorice is highly beneficial in the treatment of peptic ulcer. He says that numerous studies have attributed liquorice root with formidable antiulcer properties. For instance, Scandinavian scientists found that liquorice compounds reduced acids, stimulated mucus secretion and helped stomach wall cells repair themselves.

Pharmaceutical companies have even developed a drug called Caved-S which is essentially liquorice without its most troublesome ingredient, glycrrhizin. In a British test of 100 ulcer patients, the liquorice drug, which is chewed, was just as effective as the commonly used ulcer drug Tagamet in healing ulcers.

Liquorice is especially useful for the removal of pain caused by stomach ulcers. The demulcent action of this condiment decreases the irritation due to acids. Pieces of the dry root soaked overnight in water and the infusion taken with rice gruel greatly helps in treating ulcers.

• Cancer

Liquorice is an anti-cancer food. It has the properties, which not only help prevent cancer but also retard its spread. Triterpenoids contained in liquorice may block quick-growing cancer cells and cause some pre-cancerous cells to return to normal growth. This spice can be used either in the form of powder, decoction or infusion. These preparations can be taken mixed with honey.

• Sore throat

The spice is an effective remedy for sore throat. A small piece of raw liquorice should be chewed or sucked in treating this condition. The healing property of this spice helps cure this condition.

• Cough

Liquorice is useful in cough, where there is no phlegm. A little liquorice should be boiled in water and strained. A teaspoon of this decoction should be mixed with equal quantity of honey and taken thrice daily to obtain relief.

• Constipation

This spice is a laxative food. Thus its use has been found beneficial in the treatment of constipation. Its powder should be taken with jaggery and water.

• Muscular pains

This well-known spice possesses pain killing activity. It has been found especially helpful in muscular pains. An infusion should be prepared by soaking the dry roots overnight in water. This infusion should be given to the patients suffering from muscular pains. It is also very useful in chronic joint problems. It serves as cortisone in treating these conditions.

• Mouth disorders

Liquorice brings quick relief in tongue and mouth inflammations. The sticks should be soaked in water and the infusion used as a gargle. Tiny bits of the stick with sugar-candy can also be sucked. The demulcent action of liquorice heals the inflamed lining of the mouth and tongue.

• Baldness

Liquorice is valuable in patchy baldness where it is not due to hereditary factors. Small pieces of the root should be ground in milk with a pinch of saffron to get a paste. This paste should be heated in coconut oil, till charred and applied over the bald patches every night before going to bed. The hair grows within a few weeks. This prescription can be used when baldness has just commenced and in excessive falling of hair and dandruff with good results.

• Wounds and scalds

Liquorice powder, mixed with butter or ghee and honey, can be applied on cuts and wounds with beneficial results. The leaves of the plant, applied as a poultice, are useful in scalds of the head.

• Corns

This spice is beneficial in the treatment of corns, which are just appearing. A paste made by grinding liquorice sticks and mixing it with sesame oil or mustard oil should be rubbed into the hardened skin at bedtime. The skin gradually softens and the corn decreases in size.

Uses

Liquorice can be chewed or sucked or it can be taken in the form of powder mixed with honey or powdered jaggery. It can also be taken in the form of decoction or an infusion.

Precautions

Continuous and uninterrupted use of liquorice as a treatment for stomach ulcer is not advisable as it may cause increase in weight and puffiness of body. It should be avoided in pregnancy and in heart and kidney conditions. Eating too much liquorice can be dangerous, as it raises blood pressure.

Long Pepper

20

A Mucus-Clearing Food

Description

Long pepper *(Piper longum)* is a small, slender, trailing or climbing aromatic plant, with perennial woody roots and thin and erect branches. The leaves are seven-ribbed, smooth, 5 to 9 cm. long and 3 to 5 cm. wide. They are of two kinds. The upper leaves are oblong, egg-shaped, narrow pointed, often unequal-sided, all dark green and shining, and lower leaves are egg-shaped, equal-sided and stalked. The plant has minute flowers, small berries, 2.5 to 4 cm. egg-shaped, oblong, shiny and red in colour, when ripe. Long pepper consists of the dried fruits of the plant.

The trade name long pepper is based on the common English name pepper. It is called long pepper as its spikes are long and can be distinguished from the other important species of the genus, P. nigrum L., whose fruits are round.

Origin and distribution

Long pepper is indigenous to India. In some early literature long pepper is referred to by the name 'Magadhi' which denotes that the plant is indigenous to the region of Magadh i.e. North Bihar. It occurs in the hotter parts of India from central Himalayas to Assam, kashi and Mikir hills, lower hills of Bengal and ever-green forests of the Western Ghats from Konkan to Travancore. It also occurs in Nicobar islands. It is cultivated extensively in many places of Tamil Nadu, West Bengal and Assam, especially Cherrapunji regions which receives very heavy rains from the end of March to the Middle of September and where humidity is relatively high.

Composition

Long pepper contains alkaloids, piperine 4-5 percent and piplartine m.p. 124-250. It also contains resin and a volatile oil. The dried fruit of long pepper on steam distillation gave 0.7 percent of an essential oil of spicy odour resembling that of pepper and ginger oils.

Medicinal Virtues

The fruits have a pungent pepper-like taste and produce salivation and numbness of the mouth. Besides fruits, the roots and thicker parts of stem are cut and dried and used as an important drug in Ayurvedic and Unani medicines. The fruits as well as the roots have numerous medicinal uses.

The dried fruit is a cardiac stimulant, laxative, antiseptic and a digestive tonic. It relieves flatulence, corrects disordered

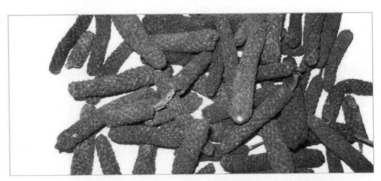

Long pepper is a cardiac stimulant, laxative, antiseptic
and a digestive tonic

processes of nutrition and restores the normal function of the system. It also allays irritation of the skin and alleviates swelling and pain and strengthens stomach.

The dried root, known as *pipal mul*, possesses some of the medicinal properties of the berries, but to an inferior degree. It is bitter and a digestive tonic. It increases the secretion and discharge of urine, strengthens the stomach and promotes its action. It also promotes sexual desire.

• Digestive disorders

Long pepper is highly beneficial in the treatment of digestive disorders like indigestion, dyspepsia, flatulence, colic and cholera. It should be given in doses of three to five decigrams, mixed with honey.

• Respiratory system disorders

This spice is a mucus-clearing food, and is therefore useful in several respiratory system disorders such as cold, cough, bronchitis, chest afflictions and asthma. It should be applied locally as counter-irritant and analgesic, and taken internally in similar manner and in same doses as for digestive disorders. A decoction of immature fruits and roots can also be used in chronic bronchitis, cough and cold.

• Rheumatic afflictions

Long pepper is an anti-inflammatory food. It has thus been found beneficial in the treatment of rheumatism and gout. Besides taking internally, it can be applied locally as a liniment. It will help relieve muscular pains and inflammation.

• Nervous disorders

The spice acts as a sedative in nervous system disorders like insomnia, epilepsy, convulsions and hysteria. It should be taken in doses of three to five decigrams mixed with honey.

• Women's problems

Long pepper is also useful in several problems concerning women. It helps promote menstruation and regulates the menstrual periods. It helps bring on abortion. It is also an efficacious remedy to check haemmorrhage and fever after childbirth.

• Other diseases

Long pepper is beneficial in the treatment of several other diseases such as fever, abdominal enlargements, leprosy, gonorrhoea and piles.

Uses

The fruits are used as spice and also preserved as pickles. In Chotta Nagpur, the root of the plant is used to ferment beer. In Andaman islands, the leaves are chewed as betel leaves.

Marjoram

21

A Household Remedy for Cold

Description

There are many varieties of Marjoram *(Majorana hortensis)* but the two most widely used for culinary purposes are the sweet or knotted Marjoram, and wild Marjoram or Oregano. Sweet Marjoram is one of the most useful spice for cooking purposes. Its flavour is to some extent similar to basil and its aroma resembles both mint and cloves.

Sweet marjoram is an aromatic plant of the mint family, which grows upto 30 to 60 cm high. Though a perennial plant, it is grown as an annual. The whole leaves are small with hairs on both sides. The flowers are tiny, green, forming small branched heads, which look like knots. Drying in the shade obtains more aromatic and less broken leaves, with less impurities.

Origin and distribution

Marjoram is a native of Southern Europe. Man's knowledge of this spice goes back to the days of mythology. Tradition speaks of this spice having been raised first by Venus, who took it from the waters of the vast ocean to the top of the highest mountain, where it was closest to the dynamic rays of the sun. Its generic name, Origanum, means 'joy of the mountains'. In Egypt it was dedicated to the Sun-God Osiris and it was offered on the altars of Greek and Roman temples. This spice is now cultivated in Western Asia, South and North America, France, Germany, England and many other countries.

Nutritive value/Composition

An analysis of the dry Marjoram shows it to contain moisture 7 percent; protein 14.31 percent; fixed oil 5.60 percent; volatile oil 1.72 percent; pentosans 7.68 percent; fibre 22.06 percent; ash 9.69 percent; tannin-an astringent substance, and ursolic acid (0.21 percent in tops; 0.05 percent in stem) are present.

Fractional distillation of the leaves and flowering heads yield a volatile oil, known as oil of sweet marjoram. However, the yield from the fresh herb is less than that from the dried herb. The oil is colourless or pale yellow to yellow-green, with a persistent odour resembling nutmeg and mint.

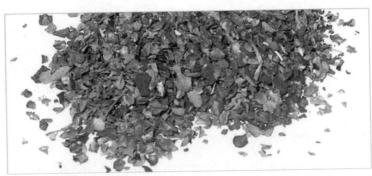

Marjoram is a stimulant and a tonic

Medicinal virtues

Greek physicians used Marjoram extensively both internally and externally. It is a stimulant and a tonic. Its flowers and seeds are useful in arresting secretion or bleeding.

• Common cold

Marjoram, with its warmth accumulated from the sun, is valuable in common cold. A tea made from this spice may be taken to treat this condition. If taken in small quantities, it stimulates the sweat glands and helps moisten, taut and dry skin during influenza.

• Headache

This spice is beneficial in the treatment of Marjoram headache. An infusion of the leaves taken as a tea relieves nervous headaches and induces sleep.

• Rheumatic afflictions

The use of Marjoram has been found effective in Rheumatic diseases. Hot fomentations of the dried leaves and tops applied in bags is helpful in relieving painful swellings and rheumatism.

• Asthma

This spice is a mucus clearing food and thus highly beneficial in the treatment of Asthma. It helps expel and loosen phlegm from the mucous membranes and the nasal and bronchial passages.

• Digestive disorders

Marjoram is valuable in digestive disorders. It expels gas from the stomach. Hot fomentations of the dried leaves and tops applied in bags is helpful in colic. The oil of marjoram can be used beneficially as hot fomentation in acute diarrhoea.

• Women's ailments

Marjoram is useful in promoting and regulating menstruation. It should be taken in the form of an infusion. This infusion also helps in promoting the secretion and flow of milk in nursing mothers.

• Skin disorders

The oil of marjoram is beneficial in the treatment of skin disorders. It can be applied externally in case of sprains, bruises, stiff and paralytic limbs. It also allays toothache.

Uses

The fresh or dried leaves of Marjoram are used fresh or dried and highly esteemed as a condiment for seasoning food. They are also used as a poultry-seasoning. Fresh leaves can be used as salad. They can also be used as garnish.

Mint

An Excellent Appetizer

22

Description

Mint *(Mentha arvensis)* is a popular spice, used extensively in Indian cooking. It is an erect, branched perennial plant upto about 60 cm. high. The shoots produced from these stems are four-angled, and bear oval-shaped leaves which are 5 cm. long, simple, delicate, thin, dark green in colour and fragrant. The flowers are small, lilac, in small bunches and are borne on axils of leaves.

The leaves have a strong, pungent odour and taste mildly bitter. They have acrid taste both in raw and cooked form. The leaves can be well-mixed with other mild tasting leaves and herbs. The leaves can also be used in the form of juice extracted from seven to 10 gms of leaves.

Origin and distribution

Mint is a native of temperate Europe. The Romans and Greeks knew about this plant from ancient times. In olden days, it was believed that Mentha, the damsel lover of God Pluto, was transferred into this plant due to the anger of Prosarpain, the wife of Pluto and Goddess of Wealth. Therefore, mint is commonly known as Mentha in Latin.

The ancient Greek physician, Saufarsats used it in the preparation of various carminative medicines. Even Mohammadan physicians were familiar with this spice. The Chinese and Japanese knew it and used it as long as two thousand years ago. Mint has now been introduced in all parts of the world and is widely grown in Indonesia, West Africa and throughout the tropics.

Mint is tolerant to a wide range of climate and soil conditions. However, it prefers a sandy loam and loam soils rich with organic matter and with good drainage. It grows well at all altitudes upto 3,500 ft. It grows throughout the year. In India, mint is grown widely in a number of varieties in Himalayan Plains and Kashmir Valley.

Nutritive value/Composition

Mint contains plenty of vitamins and is rich in several minerals. An analysis of mint leaves shows them to contain moisture 84.9 percent, protein 4.8 percent, fat 0.6 percent, minerals 1.9 percent, fibre 2.0 percent and carbohydrates 5.8 percent per 100 grams. Their mineral and vitamin contents are calcium 200 mg. percent, phosphorus 62 mg. percent, iron 15.6 mg. percent, carotene 1620 meg. percent, thiamine 0.05 mg. percent, riboflavin 0.26 mg. percent, niacin 1.0 mg. percent and vitamin C 27 mg. percent per 100 grams. They are also a rich source of vitamin D and E. Their calorific value is 48.

A golden yellow volatile oil is obtained on steam distillation of mint leaves and flowering tops. About 50 percent of menthol can be separated out in crystalline form on cooling this oil. The remaining oil is used as peppermint oil. The natural oil yields on an average 40-50 percent menthol and 50-60 percent dementholised oil which can be used both in

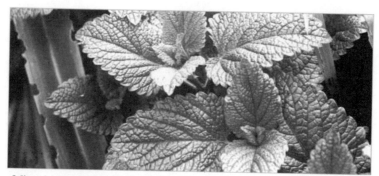

Mint is good for liver and helps dissolve gravel in the kidneys.

confectionery and medicine in place of imported peppermint oil. The dementholised oil has been found to contain menthyl acetate 24.4 percent, free menthol 44.8 percent, menthone 24.6 percent and hydrocarbons 6.2 percent. The hydrocarbons include alpha-pinene, alpha-1-limonene, carophyllene and cademene.

Medicinal virtues

Mint is much valued as a stimulant and as a drug, which relieves flatulence. It is useful in strengthening the stomach and promoting its action and also in counteracting spasmodic disorders. It forms an ingredient of most drugs prescribed for stomach ailments because of its digestive properties. It is good for the liver and helps dissolve gravel in the kidneys and bladder.

Mint oil is official in the Indian Pharmacopoeia as a carminative. It is official in the Chinese pharmacopeia as an aromatic flavoring agent, and carminative, for application to the skin and to relieve pain or discomfort. In Germany, it is taken internally as a carminative, inhaled as a secretolytic, and applied externally for its cooling property.

• Digestive system disorders

Mint is an excellent appetizer. Its fresh leaf-juice is beneficial in the treatment of indigestion, billiousness, flatulent colic, thread worms and morning sickness. It should be given mixed with a teaspoon of lime juice and honey thrice daily.

According to father Kneipp, a well-known naturopath, "A cup of mint tea, taken every morning and evening assists the digestion and gives a fresh and healthy appearance. The powder renders the same service, if one or two pinches are taken daily in the food or in water. He also considers that mint, prepared in milk or tea and drunk warm, removes abdominal pains.

The seeds of mint are beneficial in relieving abdominal gripe due to indigestion in older children. The child may be given a quarter teaspoon of the seeds to chew and swallow with water in these conditions.

Mint possesses anti-gas activity. The juice extracted from the leaves is a good appetizer. Its value is greatly enhanced by mixing equal amount of honey and lemon juice each. This mixture forms a very effective remedy for indigestion and gaseous distension of the stomach.

• Diarrhoea

Mint is an anti-diarrhoeal food. The juice extracted from this plant has been found beneficial in the treatment of diarrhoea. One teaspoon of fresh mint juice, mixed with a teaspoon each of lime juice and honey, can be given thrice daily with excellent results in the treatment of this disease.

• Respiratory disorders

Mint is valuable in respiratory disorders like tuberculosis, asthma and bronchitis. A teaspoon of fresh mint juice, mixed with two teaspoons of pure malt vinegar and equal quantity of honey stirred in 120 ml. of carrot juice, can be given thrice daily as a medicated-tonic during the treatment of these diseases. It liquefies the sputum, nourishes the lungs, increases body resistance against infection and prevents harmful effects of anti-tubercular drugs. It prevents asthmatic attacks and reduces congestion in air passages.

• Oral disorders

The fresh leaves of mint, chewed daily, is an effective antiseptic dentrifice. The chlorophyll combined with other antiseptic chemicals in the mint, kills all the harmful odour-causing germs. It strengthens the gums by providing the required nutrients and thus prevents tooth decay, pyorrhoea and pre-mature fall of the teeth. It also keeps the mouth fresh and improves the sense of taste in the tongue.

• Hoarseness

Gargling fresh mint decoction with salt has been found benefical in the treatment of hoarseness caused by shouting or singing loudly. It keeps the voice clear if used before singing. It is thus a boon to singers and orators.

• Skin disorders

The use of fresh mint juice has been found beneficial in the treatment of pimples and in the prevention of dryness of the skin. This juice should be applied externally over the affected areas. The juice can also be applied over insect stings, eczema, scabies and contact dermatitis with beneficial results.

• Dysmenorrhoea

Mint has been considered valuable in spasmodic

dysmenorrhoea or painful menstruation, especially in young girls. A tea made from it should be given for four days earlier to the expected menstrual period for treating this condition.

• Natural birth control

In Ayurveda, powdered dry mint is regarded as a harmless herb for birth control. It is believed that the women who swallows 10 grams of this powder a little before the sexual intercourse will be free from pregnancy so long as she continues this practice. The mint should be dried in a shady place and then powdered and bottled.

Uses

Mint is very popular for use in the preparation of mint and coriander *chutney*. It is also used for flavouring meat, fish, sauces, soups, stews, vinegar, teas, tobacco and cordials. The fresh leaf tops are used in beverages, apple sauces, ice-creams, jellies, salads, sauces for fish and meat. Mint oil is used in chewing gum, tooth paste and in confectionery and pharmaceutical preparations.

Mustard Seeds

A Remedy for Pains

23

Description

The mustard *(Brassica juncea)* is a well-known oil seed. It is a small annual plant, which grows upto a height of one meter with some branches. It has round stem with long internodes, simple, alternate and very soft yellowish-green leaves, about 10 cm. long and 5 cm. broad. The fruit is a pod about 2.5 cm. long, containing seeds.

There are over 150 species of mustard. Several of these species are cultivated as oilseed crops or as vegetable or fodder crops. The seeds of only three of these species namely rape, sarson and toria have condiment value.

Dry mustard seeds are small, measuring about 1 mm. in diameter. They are round and darkish-brown or greyish-brown in colour. The covering of the seeds is pitted, but the internal part is yellowish and fatty. They have no smell, but when pounded or moistured with water, they emit a peculiar pungent odour. The taste of the mustard seed is bitter and pungent.

Mustard paste is made by grinding the seeds of the black mustard and white mustard plants. In this country, mixture of the two types is used along with turmeric to give colour and wheat flour to absorb the essential oils and retard fermentation. White mustard seed is three times the size of the black seed but has less pungency and aroma. When mixed with cold water, vinegar or oil, the enzymes in the ground mustard flour produce the volatile mustard oil with its pungent smell and taste. The use of hot water or milk would destroy the enzymes and result in mustard lacking flavour.

Origin and distribution

Mustard is a native of Europe, Asia and North America. It has been in cultivation in Europe for a long time. This was the first species to provide table mustard for use as a condiment. It has been used by the Greeks, Romans and Indians from ancient times. The plant is cultivated as a field crop in most temperate countries.

Nutritive value/Composition

An analysis of mustard seed shows it to consist of moisture 8.5 percent, protein 27.0 percent, fat 39.7 percent, minerals 4.2 percent, fibre 1.8 percent and carbohydrates 23.8 percent per 100 grams. Its mineral and vitamin contents are calcium 490 mg. percent, phosphorous 700 mg. percent, iron 17.9 mg. percent, carotene 162 meg. percent, thiamine 0.65 mg. percent, riboflavin 0.26 mg. percent and niacin 4.0 mg. percent per 100 grams. Its calorific value is 541.

Black mustard seeds contain a glycoside named Sinigrin (potassium myronate) and an enzyme, Myrosin. When mustard seeds are mixed with water sinigrin and myrosin, allyl isothiocynate a volatile oil is formed. This oil is responsible for pungent, bitter smell and taste. White mustard contains a different crystalline glycoside, sinalbin along with myrosin, which combines with water and hydrolyses the sinalbin producing *acrinyl isothiocynate, sinapine acid sulphate and dextrose.* The volatile oil *acrinyl isothiocynate* is a yellow liquid that is pungent and counter irritant in its action. White mustard seeds contain 30 percent of a fixed oil, 25 percent of protein and mucillage.

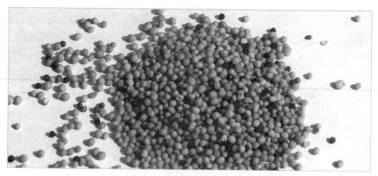

Mustard seed is antibacterial and decongestant

Medicinal Virtues

Mustard leaves have strong, hot flavour and mustard greens are an old favourite as an ingredient of soups to help clear the blood. Mustard seeds are used in condiments from time immemorial by Romans, Greeks and Indians. Pilani a physician of ancient Rome writes: It is so pungent in flavour that it burns like fire, though at the same time it is remarkably wholesome for the body'.

Mustard seed is antibacterial and decongestant. It revs up metabolism, burning off extra calories. In one British test about three-fifths of a teaspoon of ordinary yellow mustard increased metabolic rate about 25 percent, burning 45 more calories in three hours.

• Muscular pains

Mustard is a rubefacient. Its plaster or paste made with water, is applied as an analgestic in rheumatism, sciatica, paralysis of limbs and other muscular pains. The plaster should, however, never be directly applied to the skin as it may cause painful blistering. A layer of linen material should be put between the mustard paste and the skin.

• Respiratory disorders

Mustard seeds have been recognized for centuries as a decongestant and an expectorant. They help break up mucus in air passages. They are thus an effective remedy for congestion caused by colds and sinus problems. One reason why mustard seeds are mucus clearing food is that it constitutes a hot food. Mustard plasters and Mustard foot-baths, made from powdered mustard seeds are famous old age remedies for head colds and inflammation of the chest.

During an attack of asthma and bronchitis, mustard seed oil, mixed with little camphor, should be massaged over the back of the chest. This will loosen up phlegm and ease breathing. The patient should also inhale steam from the boiling water mixed with mustard and caraway seeds. It will dilate the bronchial passage.

• Poisoning

Mustard seeds have emetic properties. A teaspoon of the seeds, mixed in a glass of water, generally produces free vomiting in 5 to 10 minutes. This is especially useful in drunkenness, narcotic and other poisonings.

• Menstrual disorders

Sitz bath with mustard powder is found to be very effective in painful menstruation and scanty or stoppage of menstruation caused by exposure to cold.

• Convulsion in children

Mustard seeds are beneficial in the treatment of convulsions in children. A teaspoon of powdered mustard seeds should be mixed in five liters of warm water and it should be used as therapeutic bath in treating this condition.

• Ringworm

A paste made from mustard seeds and water has been found valuable in ringworm. This paste should be applied externally over the affected parts after washing the skin with sufficient hot water.

• Beauty aid

White mustard seeds can be used beneficially as a beauty aid. A handful of these seeds are roasted in a little sesame or coconut oil. The oil is then strained and cooled. This oil is applied with little water over face before going to bed. It will help cure pimples and whiten the complexion.

Mustard oil boiled with henna leaves is useful in healthy growth of hair. About 250 grams of mustard oil should be boiled in a tinned vessel. A little quantity of henna leaves should be gradually put in this oil till about 60 grams of these leaves are thus burnt in the oil. The oil should then be filtered through a cloth and stored well in a bottle. Regular massage of the head with this oil will produce abundant hair.

Uses

Mustard is used all over the world as an appetizer, a flavouring agent and a food preservative. The whole mustard seeds are used in pickles and chutneys. The oil extracted from the seeds is used in North India as a hair oil, oil for frying and other cooking purposes. It is also used in pickles and salads. In Punjab, Delhi and Western Uttar Pradesh, the leaves are used as a vegetable.

Nutmeg

24

An Excellent Tonic

Description

Nutmeg *(Mynistica fragrans),* a popular condiment, is the dried seed or kernel of the fruit which resembles a small peach and splits when it ripens. It is egg-shaped, approximately 2.25 to 2.75 cm. long, 1.75 to 2.25 cm. in diameter, and longitudinally wrinkled. The colour is grayish brown, with the furrows sometimes white because of lining.

Nutmeg grows on an evergreen tree, which is aromatic. It is usually nine to 12 m. high but sometimes attains a height of 20 meters or more. It has a greyish-brown smooth bark, abounding in a yellow juice. The branches spread in whorls. The leaves are alternate, elliptical, smooth aromatic, dark green and 10 to 15 cm. long and flowers are small in axillary racemes. The tree does not bloom till it is nine years old. When it fruits, it continues to do so for seventy-five years without attention.

Origin and distribution

Nutmeg is indigenous to Molucca Islands. It grows in Indonesia, Malaysia, Sri Lanka and the West Indies. It is now cultivated on a small scale in Tamil Nadu (Nilgiris), Kerala, Assam and other states. As early as the 16th century,

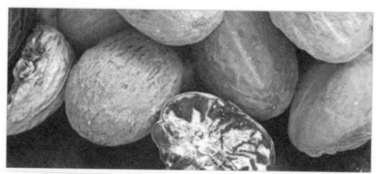

Nutmeg an effective remedy for insomnia & mental irritability

Garcoa de Oria, a Portugese physician found nutmeg trees growing luxuriantly in the Indian soil. But at present these are not found in abundance.

Nutritive value/Composition

An analysis of the nutmeg shows it to consist of moisture 14.3 percent, protein 7.5 percent, ether extract 36.4 percent, carbohydrate 28.5 percent, fibre 11.6 percent and mineral matter 1.7percent. Its mineral and vitamin contents are calcium mg 0.12 percent, phosphorus 0.24 mg percent and iron 4.6 mg. percent, thiamine 0.33 mg percent, riboflavin 0.01 mg percent and niacin 1.4 mg percent per 100 grams. Its calorific value is 472.

The nutmeg also contains an essential oil and saponin. The dry ripe seeds of the fruit contain five to 15 percent of a volatile oil and 25 to 40 percent of a fixed oil. The dry leaves of the tree yield essential oil consisting of myristica. Oil of nutmeg is a mobile almost colourless or pale yellow liquid with the characteristic odour. On ageing, it partly resinifies and becomes viscous.

Medicinal virtues

Nutmeg was used in the preparations of various medicines

in Ancient times. Even today it is officially used in several important and widely used pharmacological preparations. The oil extracted from the spice is an antispasmodic carminative.

• Digestive disorders

A mixture of 5 to 15 grams of powdered nutmeg, apple juice or banana, is used as a specific remedy for diarrhoea due to indigestion. The same quantity of powder of nutmeg, taken with a tablespoon of fresh amla juice thrice daily, is a useful medicine for indigestion, hiccup and morning sickness.

• Insomnia

The powder of nutmeg, mixed with fresh amla juice, is an effective medicine for insomnia, mental irritability and depression. Nutmeg paste mixed with honey is given as a sleeping medicine to those infants who keep on crying the whole night without any obvious reason. It should, however, not be given regularly without medical advice as it may cause serious complications and addiction.

• Sexual weakness

Nutmeg, mixed with honey and a half-boiled egg, makes an excellent sex tonic. It prolongs the duration of sexual act if taken an hour before conjugal union.

• Dehydration

This spice is useful in dehydration caused by vomiting and diarrhoea, particularly in cholera. An infusion prepared from half a nutmeg in half a litre of water should be given along with tender coconut water in doses of 15 grams at a time in treating this condition.

• Skin disorders

Nutmeg is beneficial in the treatment of skin diseases like ringworm and eczema. A paste of the spice, made by rubbing it on a stone slab, in one's own early morning saliva before cleaning the mouth, is applied once daily as a specific medicine in the treatment of these conditions.

• Rheumatic pains

A nutmeg coarsely powdered and fried in til oil until all the particles become brown, is very useful as an external application to relieve rheumatic pains, neuralgia and sciatica. The oil should be cooled and strained before application.

• Common cold

In case of a running nose, paste made from this spice and cow's milk together with 75 mg. of opium should be applied to the forehead and the nose. It will provide quick relief.

• Beneficial effect on the eyes

Nutmeg exercises beneficial effect on the eyes. A paste of this spice made with milk may be applied all around the eyes and over the eyelids. It will have cooling effect.

Uses

Nutmeg is used as a condiment and in medicine. Oil of nutmeg is employed for flavouring food products and liquor. It is also used in liniments, perfumery and hair lotions.

Precautions

Nutmeg should be taken in very small doses as in large doses, it excites the motor cortex and produces epileptic convulsions and lessions in the liver. Even a teaspoon of nutmeg can produce toxic symptoms such as burning in the stomach, nausea, vomiting, restlessness, giddiness with fear of death and feeling of great excitement.

Onion

25

Dynamite of Natural Foods

Description

Onion *(Allium cepa)* is one of the most important vegetable and a condiment crop grown all over India. It has characteristic flavour, which accounts for its popularity. It is the pungent edible bulb of the lily family, and one of the oldest cultivated crops. It is considered a food of exceptional value for flavouring and seasoning.

The onion is a hardy, bulbous, biennial plant, usually grown as an annual. It has superficial root system, a very short flattened stem at the base of the plant, which increases in diameter as growth continues. The leaves of the plant are long, linear, hollow and cylindrical. A bulb is formed by thickening of the leaf bases when the plant reaches a certain stage of growth. The fruit is a round capsule. Bulbs have a pungent and overpowering odour. All the parts of the plant produce a strong onion odour when crushed.

Origin and distribution

Onion is believed to have originated in Central Asia, possibly in the Iran-Pakistan region. It has been cultivated since ancient times in the Middle East and India. It was a popular food in ancient Egypt, where it is depicted on tombs as early as 3,200 B.C. It was eaten by the builders of the pyramids, and was used in religious and funerary offerings. It has been found in mummies.

The Sanskrit word for onion is *palandu,* which has been mentioned in the *Garuda Purana.* The great Indian sages, Maharishi Atreya and Lord Dhanwantri have described the use of onions in details. It is referred to in the Bible and the Koran. It is frequently mentioned in the literature from Hippocrates, 430 B.C. down to the present time.

Onion was introduced into the New World shortly after its discovery, and was cultivated there as early as 1629. It has now spread to most parts of the World. The most important onion-growing states in India are Maharashtra, Andhra Pradesh, Tamil Nadu, Bihar and Punjab.

Nutritive value/Composition

Onion has been described as the dynamite of natural foods. Compared with other fresh vegetables, it is relatively high in food value, moderate in protein content and is rich in calcium and riboflavin. There is considerable variation in composition between different varieties and it also varies with stage of maturity and the length of storage.

An analysis of a mature onion shows its content as moisture 86.6 percent, protein 1.2 percent, fat 0.1 percent, fibre 0.6 percent, minerals 0.4 percent and carbohydrate 11.1 percent per 100 grams of edible portion. The carbohydrate is principally in the form of sugars. Its mineral and vitamin contents are calcium 47 mg. percent, phosphorus 50 mg. percent, iron 0.7 mg. percent, carotene 15 meg. percent, thiamine 0.08 mg. percent, riboflavin 0.01 mg. percent, niacin 0.4 mg. percent per 100 grams. Its calorific value is 51.

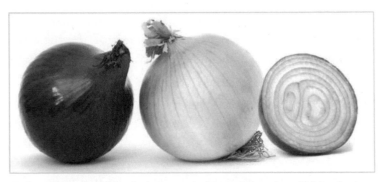

Onion thins the blood, lowers cholesterol, wards off blood clots
and fights asthma and diabetes.

The bulbs and fresh herb yield 0.005 percent of an essential
oil which has an acrid taste and unpleasant odour. The chief
constituent of the crude oil is allyl-propyl disulphide. The
odour in onion is due to organic sulphur compounds, and is
produced only when the tissues are cut or injured by enzyme
action on the water-soluble amino acid. Heat or freeze drying
prevents the enzyme action, so that cooking produces a
different odour, flavour and pungency. The pungent flavour
of onions is much appreciated by many people in many
countries.

Medicinal virtues

Onion is one of civilizations oldest medicines. It was
reputed in ancient Mesopotamia to cure virtually every
disease. The physicians of ancient Egypt prescribed onions
in various diseases. Dioscorides in the first century A.D.
attributed many herbal remedies to them. They are
stimulant, diuretic, expectorant and rubefacient. Onions
should be taken with meals, preferably raw, as fried or
cooked onions are comparatively difficult to digest. For
therapeutic purposes, it is advisable to use onion juice instead
of the whole onion as it is an all-round medicine.

An exceptionally strong antioxidant, onion is full of numerous anticancer compounds. It has been specifically linked to inhibit human stomach cancer. It thins the blood, lowers cholesterol, raises good-type HDL cholesterol, wards off blood clots, and fights asthma, chronic bronchitis, hay fever, diabetes, atherosclerosis and infections.

The leaves of the plant are diuretic, carminative, digestive, emmolient, tonic, alterative, anthelmintic, stimulant, expectorant, antispasmodic, mild laxative and aphrodisiac.

• Respiratory disease

Onion is a mucus clearing food. It liquefies phlegm and prevents its further formation. It has been used as a food remedy for centuries in cold, cough, bronchitis and influenza. Equal amounts of onion juice and honey should be mixed and three to four teaspoons of this mixture should be taken daily in treating these conditions. It is one of the safest preventive medicines against common cold during winter.

• Tooth disorders

Latest researches have confirmed the bactericidal properties of onion. According to these findings, if a person consumes one raw onion every day by thorough mastication, he will be protected from a host of tooth disorders. The Russian Doctor, BP. Tohkin, who has contributed to this research, has expressed the opinion that chewing raw onion for three minutes is sufficient to kill all the germs in the mouth. Toothache is often allayed by placing a small piece of onion on the bad tooth or gum.

• Heart disease

Onion is regarded as preventive against heart attack. It has been found helpful and beneficial in diseases of the heart. These benefits are due to the presence of essential oil, allypropyl disulphide, catechol, protocatechnic acid, thiopropiono aldehyde, thiocyanate, Ca, P, Fe and vitamins.

• Sexual impotence

Onions have been attributed aphrodisiac properties since prehistoric times. They have been hailed as more than foods in the Egyptian, Greek, Roman, Arab and Chinese literature. A 16th century Arabic erotic manual called *The Perfumed Garden* written by Sheikh Al Nefzawi, recommends use of the juice of pounded onions mixed with honey to improve sexual power. Onions were considered so potent that in olden times celibate Egyptian priests were prohibited from eating them. This vegetable is believed to increase libido and strengthen the reproductive organ. In France, newly-weds were fed onion soup in the morning after their wedding night to restore their libido.

A syrup made from onion and honey has been found very effective in restoring sexual power. This syrup is prepared by mixing 30 grams of onion juice with 60 grams of honey and placing it on fire. It should be taken off the fire when it obtains the consistency of syrup. A person may take even double the dose, if it suits him. It reddens the face within a few days and is one of the best aphrodisiac foods.

• Skin disorders

Onion is irritating to the skin and stimulates the circulation of blood in the mucous membrane. Warts also sometimes disappear when rubbed with cut onions. Roasted onions are applied as a poultice to indolent boils, bruises and wounds to relieve heating sensation and bring the boils to maturity.

• Diabetes

Onions have been used as a treatment for diabetes since ancient times. Research studies conducted have proved that this pungent vegetable can lower blood sugar in diabetes. Research scientist fed subjects onion juice and whole onions in doses of 25 to 200 grams and found that the greater the dose, the more the blood sugar decrease. It makes no difference whether the onion was eaten in raw or cooked form. The investigators found that the onions affect the liver's metabolism of glucose, or release of insulin, or prevent insulin's destruction.

The probable active hypoglycemic substances in onions are allyl proply disulphide and allicin. In fact, as early as 1923, researchers had detected blood-sugar-lowering property in onion. And in the 1960s, scientist isolated anti-diabetic compounds from onions, which are similar to the common anti-diabetic pharmaceuticals that are used to release and stimulate insulin synthesis.

• High blood cholesterol

Onions are credited with the property to lower bad LDL cholesterol and raise good HDL type. Raw onion is one of the best treatments for boosting beneficial HDL cholesterol. According to Dr. Victor Gurewich, a cardiologist and professor of medicine at Harvard Medical School, half a raw onion, or equivalent in juice, raises HDL an average 30 percent in most people with heart disease or cholesterol problems. He, however, says that more you cook the onions, the more they lose their HDL-raising powers. The onion therapy works in about 70 percent of patients. If a person cannot eat half a raw onion a day, he may eat less. Any amount may help raise good HDL cholesterol.

• Viral diseases

Onions are an antiviral food. The Quercetin, concentrated in it, has antiviral and antibacterial activity. This condiment is thus beneficial in the treatment of several viral diseases, especially cold and influenza. The use of a hot roasted onion before retiring to bed at night is an effective remedy for common cold. For treating influenza, equal amounts of onion juice and honey should be mixed, and three or four teaspoons of this mixture should be taken daily. A French military physician, Dr. Melamet, during World War II treated the influenza patients at his hospital, at St. Servan by giving them daily the juice of pounded onions three times a day in a warm infusion. Under this treatment the temperature came down within two days and the patients who were so treated survived.

Onions are also valuable in warts caused by viral infection. They are irritating to the skin and they stimulate the circulation of the blood. Warts sometimes disappear when rubbed with cut onions.

• Cholera

Onion is an effective remedy for cholera. About 30 grams of onion and seven black peppers should be finely pounded in a pestle and given to the patient of cholera. It allays thirst and restlessness and the patient feels better. It also lessens vomiting and diarrhoea.

Onion can help prevent cholera infection during epidemic. It should be cut into pieces and scattered all over the house during cholera epidemic. This will prevent an attack of the diseases. A sauce prepared from onion can also be beneficially used with food during cholera epidemic, this will help prevent the disease. The method of preparing this sauce is to peel the onion and cut it into small pieces. These pieces should then be washed in a small amount of water several times. Vinegar and common salt may be added to taste. This sauce may be used with each meal. It is quite tasteful and effective against cholera.

• Ear infection

The juice extracted from an onion can be used beneficially in the treatment of pus formation in the ear caused by middle-ear infection. It should be slightly warm and put into the ear two or three times daily in treating this condition.

• Rheumatic diseases

Onion possesses anti-inflammatory activity. Its regular use, especially in raw form, can help reduce inflammation in arthritis and other rheumatic diseases. The juice of this vegetable, mixed with mustard oil in equal quantity, can also be applied externally, with beneficial results, to allay pains and swellings in rheumatic afflictions.

• Blood clots

Onions are anti-coagulant food. Eating them either in raw or cooked form, helps keep blood free of clots. Harvard's Dr. Victor Gurewich advised all his patients with coronary heart disease to eat onions daily, partly because their compounds hinder platelet clumping and increase clot dissolving activity.

In fact, onions have a truly wonderful ability to counteract the detrimental clot-promoting effects of eating fatty foods. This was shown by Dr. N.N. Gupta, professor of medicine at K.G. Medical College in Lucknow. He first fed men a very-high-fat meal, with butter and cream, and discovered that their clot-dissolving activity greatly decreased. Then he gave them the same fatty meal, this time adding 55 grams of onions, raw, boiled or fried. Blood drawn two and four hours after the fatty meal showed that the onions had totally blocked the fat's detrimental blood-clotting proclivities. In fact, 100 grams of onions completely reversed the fat's damaging effects on clot-dissolving activity.

• Aches and pains

Onion possesses pain killing property. It is beneficial in the treatment of pain in the eye. The juice of onion and honey should be mixed in equal quantity and stored in a bottle. This mixture should be applied to the eyes by means of an eye-rod. It will provide relief in a short time.

Onion is a valuable medicine for suppressing pain resulting from piles. Occasionally, blind piles swell up and cause torturous pain to the patient. It becomes extremely difficult for the patient even to sit. For treating this condition, two onions should be half-baked by burying them in live ash. They should then be thoroughly pounded into a paste after removing their outer covering. This paste should be fried in ghee and a tablet prepared from it. This tablet should be placed over the piles while hot. It should be retained there in position by applying a suitable dressing.

The patient will feel comfort immediately after this application. The patient suffering from piles should daily eat onion and caraway seeds, fried in ghee, with sugar candy. A compress made of the pulp of roasted onions should also be applied over the inflamed and protruding piles. An ointment made of onion, turmeric and Indian hemp in hot sesame oil also makes an effective application over pile masses.

• Urinary system disorders

Onion is an effective diuretic food and very beneficial in the treatment of urinary system disorders. For burning sensation with micturition, a decoction of this vegetable has proved very valuable. This decoction is prepared by boiling six grams of onions in 500 ml of water, till half of the water has evaporated. It should then be strained and taken by the patient when cold.

In urine retention, onion should be rubbed in water and 60 grams of sugar should be mixed with it. The patient should have this mixture and it will result in free urination within a short time. The effect will be greatly enhanced if a little potassium nitrate is added to this mixture.

• Dsymenorrhoea

Onion is a valuable remedy for painful menstrution. About 50 gm. of onions should be boiled in two litres of water and sugar candy added to sweeten it. This drink should be taken warm in treating this condition.

• Antioxidant

Onion is the richest dietary source of quercetin, a powerful antioxidant. This substance is found only in yellow and red onions and not in white. Some onion are so full of quercetin that the compound accounts for up to 10 percent of their dry weight, according to tests by Terrance Leighton, Ph.D., professor of biochemistry and molecular biology at the University of California at Berkeley.

Uses

Onion can be used in innumerable ways. The immature and mature bulbs are eaten raw or they may be cooked and eaten as vegetable. They are used in soups and sauces and for seasoning many foods. They may also be eaten fried. Onion oil, produced by steam distillation, is used to a limited extent for flavouring foods.

Precautions

Excessive use of onions should, however, be avoided as it may promote gas formation and aggravate heartburn. Recent experiments have also found that abundant use of onions have a tendency to reduce the number of red cells and to lower the haemoglobin.

26 Pepper

King of Spices

Description

Pepper *(Piper nirgum)* is one of the oldest and most Popular of all spices. It is known as 'King of Spices'. The pepper plant is a stout, evergreen creeper with smooth surface, much swollen at the nodes. The leaves of the plant resembles betel leaves and are broadly egg-shaped, 10 to 22 cm. long, 11 cm. broad, and leathery with five to nine ribs. The flowers are slender and they protect drooping spikes.

The fruits are berries having a pendulous spike and are borne in clusters. When the fruits are tender, they are pale or dark green in colour. As they ripen, they become red and dark purple. The berries are than separated from the stalk. Pepper berries are spherical, dark brown or black in colour and about 5 mm. in diameter. The pericarp is thin, and contains a single seed completely filling the cavity.

Black and white pepper are prepared from the berries of the same plant or species. For preparing black pepper, however, spikes are harvested when berries are fully mature, but unripe, that is when green or greenish yellow. For preparing white pepper, the harvesting of berries is delayed until they become ripe that is yellowish red or red. White pepper is prepared by removing the outer pericarp of the harvested berries, either before or after drying. Both black and white peppers are ground and used in powdered form.

Origin and distribution

Pepper is a native of western Ghats of India. It occurs wild in the hills of Assam and north Burma, but may have become naturalized in the region from an early introduction. In the 16th century, pepper was grown on the West Coast of India with Malabar as the centre. During the 20th century, this spice has been introduced into most tropical countries. Pepper is cultivated in India from the Vedic period. It was mentioned by Theophrastus in 372-287 B.C. It was used by the ancient Greeks and the Romans. By the Middle Ages, pepper had assumed great importance. It was used to season insipid food and as a preservative in curing meats. Together with other spices, it helps to overcome the odours of bad food.

Nutritive value/Composition

An analysis of black pepper shows it to consist of moisture 13.2 percent, protein 11.5 percent, fat 6.8 percent, minerals 4.4 percent, fibre 14.9 percent and carbohydrates 49.2 percent per 100 grams. Its mineral and vitamin contents are calcium 460 mg. percent, iron 198 mg. percent, phosphorus 16.8 mg. percent, carotene 1080 meg. percent, thiamine 0.09 mg. percent, riboflavin 0.14 percent and niacin 1.4 mg. percent per 100 grams. Its calorific value is 304.

An analysis of 23 types of black pepper from kerala, South and North Kanara, Coorg and Assam gave the following ranges of values; total nitrogen 1.55-2.6 percent, nitrogen in non-volatile ether extract 2.7-4.22 percent, volatile ether extract 0.3-4.2 percent, non-volatile ether extract 3.9-11.5

percent, alcohol extract 4.4-12 percent, starch 28.0-49.0 percent, crude peperine 2.8-9.0 percent and acid insol (ash) 0.03-0.55 percent. Thus, India produces numerous types of black pepper that are characterized by variations in size, colour, flavour and physico-chemical properties.

The predominant constituent of pepper is starch. It accounts for 34.8 percent in black pepper, 56.5 percent in white pepper and 63.2 percent in decorticated white pepper. Pepper starch consists of minute polygonal granules resembling those of rice, but much smaller. The hilum is visible only under high power magnification. The characteristic aromatic odour of pepper is due to the presence of a volatile oil in the cells of pericarp. On steam distillation, crushed black pepper yields 1.0 to 2.6 percent of the volatile oil.

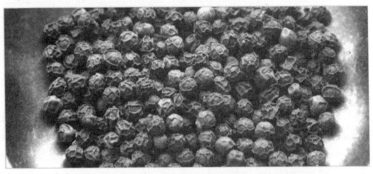

Black pepper is stimulant, pungent, aromatic, digestive and nervine tonic.

Medicinal virtues

Black pepper is a stimulant, pungent, aromatic, digestive and nervine tonic. The pungency of pepper is due to the resin chavicine, which is most abundant in the mesocarp. Black pepper is useful in relieving flatulence.

• Digestive disorders

Black pepper has stimulating action on the digestive organs

and it produces an increased flow of saliva and gastric juices. It is an appetizer and a good home remedy for digestive disorders. A quarter teaspoon of pepper powder mixed in thin buttermilk should be taken in indigestion or heaviness in the stomach. For better results, an equal part of cumin powder may also be added to the buttermilk.

• Colds

This spice is beneficial in the treatment of cold and fever. Six pepper seeds finely ground should be mixed in a glass of warm water along with six pieces of batasha. This drink should be taken for a few days every night in treating this condition. In case of acute coryza, 20 gms. pepper powder should be boiled in milk with a pinch of turmeric powder and used once daily for three days. It will bring beneficial results. About 12 roasted pepper corns, mixed with honey, can also be used beneficially in the treatment of cold and rhinitis. They should be taken once daily.

• Amnesia

A pinch of finely-ground pepper mixed with honey is useful in amnesia or dullness of intellect. It should be taken both in the morning and evening.

• Cough

Black pepper is an effective remedy for cough due to throat irritation. Three pepper corns should be chewed with a pinch of corns caraway seeds and a crystal of common salt to get relief.

• Prolapse of the rectum

This spice is beneficial in the treatment of prolapse of the

Rectum. About 30 gms. of the powder of black peppers and 20 gms. of caraway seeds should be mixed with 200 ml. of honey. About 20 ml. of this mixture should be taken daily on an empty stomach for seven days.

• Arsenic poisoning

Pepper can be used beneficially as an antidote for arsenic poisoning. About 15 gms. of pepper powder should be mixed with honey and given thrice daily for this purpose.

• Snake bite

This spice is valuable in snake bite and scorpion sting. An infusion of the peppers prepared from 20 corns in 180 ml. of water should be taken thrice daily in treating these conditions.

• Impotence

Eating six black peppers with four almonds once daily, with milk is a nerve-tonic. It acts as an aphrodisiac, especially in a young impotent person.

• Muscular pain

As an external application, pepper dilates the superficial vessels and acts as a counter-irritant. A tablespoon of pepper powder fried in sesame oil until it is charred, can be applied beneficially as an analgesic liniment for mylagia and rheumatic pains.

• Tooth disorders

The powder of pepper and common salt is an excellent dentifrice. Its daily use prevents the dental caries, foul breath, bleeding from the gums and toothache. A pinch of pepper powder mixed with clove oil, is put in the caries to alleviate toothache.

Peppers are useful in pyorrhoea or pus in the gums. Finely powdered pepper and salt mixture should be massaged over the gums. This relieves inflammation and swelling.

Uses

Pepper is most widely used as a condiment. Its flavour and pungency blend well with most savoury dishes. It has extensive culinary uses. It is used in pickles, ketchups and sauces, for seasoning dishes and in sausages.

Poppy Seeds

A Cooling Medicine

27

Description

Poppy plant *(Papaver somniferum)* is cultivated either for manufacture of opium or for poppy seeds. It is an erect, annual plant, with smooth surface and latex in all parts. It is endowed with roots of strong fragrance. The milky ooze from poppy plant obtained by incision from the unripened capsules and thickened by spontaneous evaporation, is known as opium. Opium is one of the most valuable medicines available in the sap of the plants and if properly administered, can serve as a very useful drug.

Poppy seeds are found in poppy heads. They are white in colour and very small in size. They are so small that one thousand seeds weigh only 0.25 to 0.5 gm. They are recommended in many prescriptions for tonics.

Origin and distribution

Poppy plant is a native of Asia Minor. It was known to the ancient Greeks, and reached India and China by the eighth century. The main areas of cultivation are now in India, China, Asia Minor and the Balkans.

Nutritive value/Composition

An analysis of poppy seeds shows them to consist of moisture 4.3 percent, protein 21.7 percent, fat 19.3 percent, minerals 9.9 percent, fibre 8.0 percent and carbohydrates 36.8 percent per 100 gm. Their mineral contents are calcium 1584 mg percent, phosphorus 432 mg percent and iron 15.9 mg percent per 100 gm. Its calorific value is 408.

The sap of the plant contains oxalic acid and opium. Opium has 25 alkaloids. The most important of these are morphine, codeine, thelaine, narcotine, narceine and papaverine. The seeds have a high protein content, the major component being globulin which accounts for 55 percent of the total nitrogen. The amino acid make-up of the globulin is similar to that of the whole seed protein.

Poppy seeds contain upto 50 percent of an edible oil which, is extracted by either cold or hot expression. The oil is odourless and possesses a pleasant almond-like taste. In India, the oil is generally extracted by cold-pressing the seed in small presses in homes or small establishments. Raw cold-pressed oil is pale yellow to golden yellow in colour.

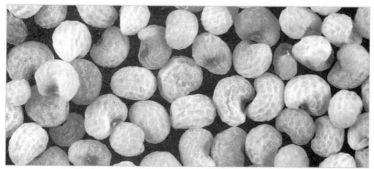

Poppy seeds are of great value as a calming and sedative food.

Medicianl virtues

Poppy seeds are effective in thirst, fever, inflammation and irritation of the stomach. The root is employed as one of the ingredients in several cooling medicines. An infusion of the root is given as a febrifuge or fever relieving drink and a powder in bilious complaints. The essence of the root is used as tonic because of its stimulating qualities. It is believed to check vomiting in cholera.

• Sleeplessness

The seeds can be beneficially used as a valuable medicine in sleeplessness. About 30 grams of milk extracted from the seeds mixed with sugar can be used for treating this condition. A teaspoon of poppy seed oil taken every night is also very effective.

• Dysentery

An easy-to-make home remedy for dysentery is to saute about a quarter teaspoon of the powder of poppy seeds to golden brown in honey. It should be taken twice a day, it will relieve the symptoms of the disease. As these seeds have a sedative effect, they should not be taken for more than three days continuously.

• Heat and burning sensation

As an external remedy, the poppy plant has many uses. A paste of the root rubbed on the skin can remove burning sensation of the body. A paste made from the pulverised roots in water can be used as a cooling agent. It can be used beneficially as an external application in fevers.

• Dry itch

Poppy seeds are valuable in dry itch. They should be ground to a paste with lime juice and rubbed on the affected areas.

• Pains and aches

Poppy seeds on the stalks, which have not been slit to produce opium have soporific properties and are used for relieving pain.

Opium is useful in rheumatism, tumours of different kinds, cancers, carbuncles, abscesses, ulcers, leprosy, syphilis or scrofula—that is, tuberculosis of the lymph node in which pain banishes sleep, especially at night. The commencing dose is 6 centigram of the extract. If it is insufficient, upto 18 centigrams may be advised to those who are unaccustomed to opium. Beyond this, it is unsafe to do so without any professional advice. This may be combined with 12 or 18 centigrams of camphor. Opium is very effective in spasms of bowels, relieving of pain and irritation of the bladder caused by stone.

Opium is useful as a liniment for soothing, both muscular and neuralgic pains. The liniment can be prepared by mixing 90 centigrams of opium in 15 grams of coconut oil. It even soothes painful piles. In painful teeth cavities, a centigram of opium is put into the hollow of the tooth. Care should, however, be taken not to swallow the saliva.

Uses

The poppy seeds are used as food and as a source of fatty oil. They are considered nutritive and used in breads, curries, sweets and confectionery.

Precuations

Opium can cause great harm if used without proper precautions, or in cases where the person is intolerant to its action or gets upset even with a smallest dose. In such cases, the drug should be avoided.

Infants and young children have poor tolerance to opium and they should be administered only under medical advice. It should be avoided during pregnancy and in kidney diseases.

28

Saffron

A Stimulant Food

Description

Saffron *(Crocus sativus)* is a bulbous perennial plant, which grows from 15-25 cm. in height. It is a low growing plant with an underground globular corn and grass-like leaves. It is cultivated for its large, scented, blue or lavender flowers. The flowers have trifid, orange coloured stigmas, which along with the style-tops yield the saffron of commerce. It has a bitter taste and a penetrating aromatic odour.

Saffron is one of the world's oldest and expensive spices. It is estimated that one pound of saffron consists of about 225,000 to 500,000 dried stigmas, and requires the picking by hand of 75,000 flowers. That gives an idea of the human labour involved in harvesting saffron.

Origin and distribution

Saffron is a native of Southern Europe. It was known to the ancient Greeks and Romans. Saffron was imported to England from the East many centuries ago, and was once grown extensively around Saffron Walden, in Essex. One smoke-pervaded spot in the heart of London still bears the name of 'Saffron Hill.' It is now cultivated in Mediterranean countries, particularly in Spain, Austria, France, Greece, England, Turkey, Persia, India and the Orient. The valley of Kashmir in India is famous for its saffron fields extending to about 3350 acres.

Nutritive value/Composition

An analysis of saffron shows it to contain on an average moisture 15.6 percent, starch and sugar 13.35 percent, essential oil 0.6 percent, fixed oil 5.63 percent, total and free extract 43.64 percent, crude fiber 4.48 percent and ash 4.27 percent per 100 gm.

The yield of essential oil and fixed oil is as high as 1.37 percent and 13.4 percent respectively. The ash is rich in potassium and phosphorus and contains traces of boron. The essential oil contains terpenes, terpene alcohols and esters. It also contains glucosides protocrocines and picrocrocines, which are the principle colouring agent and the bitter substance respectively.

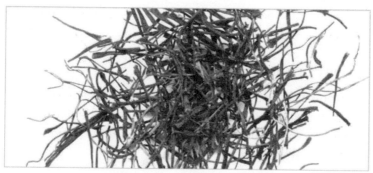

The use of Saffron has been found beneficial in treatment of fevers, melancholia, enlargement of liver and spleen.

Medicinal virtues

Saffron is credited with various medicinal properties. It is largely used in indigenous medicine across India. It is an important ingredient of the Ayurvedic and Unani system of medicine. Saffron enjoys great reputation as a drug, which strengthens the functioning of stomach and promotes its action. It also counteracts spasmodic disorders and sustains involuntary muscle contraction. It is a stimulant and promotes libido. In modern pharmacopoeias, saffron is employed only to colour other medicines or as a cordial adjunct.

• Digestive disorders

Saffron is beneficial in the treatment of several digestive disorders. Its use has been found especially valuable in flatulent colic.

• Women's ailments

This spice is useful in promoting and regulating menstrual periods. It soothes lumbar pains, which accompany menstruation. Saffron is also beneficial in the treatment of other ailments concerning women such as leucorrhoea and hysteria. Pessaries of saffron are used in painful conditions of the uterus. Saffron oil is used as an external application in uterine sores.

• Urinary disorders

Saffron has been found beneficial in the treatment of urinary problems. It should be soaked over night in water and used in the morning with honey for treating these conditions. It promotes free urination.

• Skin disorders

Saffron is useful in treating skin disorders. A paste of the spice can be used as a dressing for bruises and superficial sores.

• Other diseases

The use of this spice has been found beneficial in several other diseases. These includes, fevers, melancholia, enlargement of liver and spleen and catarrhal affections in children. When pounded with ghee, it is reported to be effective in the treatment of diabetes.

Uses

Saffron is mostly used for flavouring and colouring purposes. It is used in foreign countries in exotic dishes particularly, in Spanish rice specialities and French fish preparations. It is also used for baking bread in Scandinavia, the Balkans and many countries.

Precautions

Saffron has been employed as an abortifacient. It should therefore, not be taken in large doses by pregnant women as it may cause abortion. Saffron bulbs are toxic to young animals, and stigmas in overdose are narcotic.

Tamarind

29

An Antiseptic Food

Description

The tamarind *(Tamarindus indica)* fruit or pulp is very popular all over India as a condiment and as a souring substance. It plays an important role in numerous culinary preparations in the country, specially southern India where it constitutes an essential ingredient of sambars, rasams, chutneys and curries.

The tamarind tree is one of the important big trees, which grows upto 40 mtrs. in height. It has a broad trunk. It is an ornamental tree with a longevity of 120 years. The leaves of the tree are leguminous, 2.5 cm. long, 1.25 cm. broad and sour in taste. The flowers are yellowish with reddish streaks, in small erect clusters among the leaves and sour in taste.

Fruits are legumes measuring from 8 to 20 cm. long, 2 to 3 cm. broad, flesh, brown in colour and crescent in shape when it is tender. It is brown coloured outside, over the green epicarp. As the fruit ripens the covering becomes hard and brittle and the pulp becomes dark-maroon, having strings of fibres. The pulp is sourish-sweet in taste and emits a typical sour odour. When the outer covering is dry, the fruits are plucked and the pulp is separated from the outer covering, fibres and seeds. The seeds are dark brown and shining and they are embedded in the fleshy fibrous mass, which is the well-known acid pulp of Tamarind.

Origin and distribution

Tamarind is a native of Africa and South India. The tree is now grown in most tropical countries both for its fruits and as a shady tree. It occurs commonly in the central and southern regions of India and is planted throughout the country on roadsides and in gardens.

Nutritive value/Composition

An analysis of tamarind pulp shows it to consist of moisture 20.9 percent, protein 3.1 percent, fat 0.1 percent, minerals 2.9 percent, fibre 5.6 percent and carbohydrates 67.4 percent per 100 grams. Its mineral and vitamin contents are calcium 170 mg. percent, phosphorus 110 mg. percent, iron 10.9 mg. percent, carotene 60 meg. percent, riboflavin 0.07 mg. percent, niacin 0.7 mg. percent and vitamin C 3 mg. percent. Its calorific value is 283.

The pulp contains tartaric acid 9.8 percent, combined acid 6.8 percent, total invert sugars 38.2 percent and pectin 2.8 percent. The pectin present in pulp is of good quality having a jelly grade of 180-200.

Medicinal virtues

Tamarind was an important item of diet in the sailing ships of olden times as the acid and sugar contents of the fruit helped offset the starchy diet of seamen.

The leaves and bark of the tree as well as pulp and seeds of the fruit have medicinal virtues. The leaves are stimulant, cooling and antibilious. They also increase the secretion and discharge of urine. The bark is an astringent,

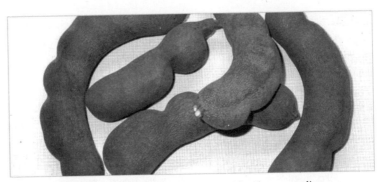

Tamarind pulp is digestive, antiflatulent, cooling, laxative and antiseptic.

and a tonic and it reduces fever. The pulp of the fruit is digestive, antiflatulent, cooling, laxative and antiseptic. The seeds are astringent.

• Digestive disorders

The pulp of the ripe fruit is beneficial in the treatment of bilious vomiting, flatulence and indigestion. It is also useful in constipation. An infusion of the pulp prepared by macerating it in water is particularly useful for loss of appetite and disinclination for food. For better results, black pepper, cloves, cardamoms and camphor to taste may be added to this infusion after straining.

For gastric problem, a mixture of a tamarind and jaggery has been found highly valuable. The method of preparing this mixture is to take some tamarind, which has been preserved for more than one year, and soak it overnight in water kept in an earthen container. It should be mixed well with a stick and strained, if necessary. Soaked tamarind and jaggery may be mixed in equal quantity with one tablespoon of lime, mixing it well again with a stick. When it becomes like jam, it should be put in a glass container, filling only three-fourths of the container. It should be closed loosely and left for 72 hours. A teaspoon of this jam should be taken twice daily on an empty stomach for 30 days.

Another method of using tamarind for the treatment of digestive problems like morning sickness, indigestion and pyrosis is to chew a piece of tamarind with some salt and pepper. This method has been used as a folk-medicine for centuries in treating these conditions. The ash obtained by heating the bark with salt in an earthen vessel can also be given in 6 to 12 centigram doses for colic and indigestion with beneficial results.

• Scurvy

Tamarind pulp, being rich in vitamin C, is valuable in preventing and curing scurvy. It is significant that tamarind does not lose its antiscorbutic property on drying as other fruits and vegetables.

• Cold

Tamarind-pepper 'rasam' is considered a food of exceptional value in clearing mucus. It is used as an effective home remedy for cold in South India. It is prepared by boiling for a few minutes very dilute tamarind water in a teaspoon of ghee and half a teaspoon of black pepper powder. This steaming hot rasam has a flushing effect. As one takes it, the nose and eyes water and the nasal blockage is cleared.

• Fevers

The pulp of tamarind fruit is useful in febrile disorders. It is generally given in 15 gram doses. A sherbet made by boiling 30 grams of the pulp in half a litre of milk with addition of few dates, cloves, sugar, cardamoms and a little camphor is an efficacious drink in fevers.

• Piles

The use of the covering of the tamarind seed has been found beneficial in the treatment of piles. This covering should be finely powdered and a pinch of the powder should be given thrice daily for a week in treating this condition.

• Burns

The tender leaves of tamarind tree are a useful remedy for treating burns. The leaves should be put into a pot, covered and warmed over the fire. The burnt leaves are finely powdered and then sieved to remove gritty particles. This fine powder should be mixed in gingelly(til) oil and applied over the burnt part. The wound will be healed within a few days. The leaves prevent oedema formation and bring about the growth of healthy normal skin. Oil being impermeable, keeps the affected part well protected against moisture and entry of harmful germs.

• Skin disorders

An infusion of the leaves can be used for washing foul-smelling ulcers. The paste of these leaves can also be applied over scabies with beneficial results. The powder of the dry leaves is dusted for treating leg ulcers and boils.

• Rhuematic afflications

The leaves of this tree are an anti-inflammatory medicine and thus highly beneficial in the prevention and treatment of arthritis, rheumatism and gout. The leaves should be crushed with water and made into a poultice. This poultice can be applied externally over the inflamed joints and ankles with beneficial results. This will reduce swelling and pain.

• Sexual disability

The use of tamarind seeds has been found beneficial in the treatment of sexual debility and dysfunction. A powder should be prepared from the seeds, after removing the outer covering by soaking them in water for 4 days. This powder should be mixed with equal quantity of sugar, powder of puffed Bengal gram, few seeds of cardamom and dates. A teaspoon of this mixture should be taken once daily with a glass of milk. This will help cure nocturnal emissions and spermatorrhoea.

• Sore throat

Tamarind water as a gargle is beneficial in the treatment of sore throat. A powder of the dry leaves can also be beneficially used as a gargle for this condition. An infusion of the bark is equally beneficial in the treatment of sore throat.

Uses

The ripe fruit or tamarind pulp is used in numerous culinary preparations notably, 'sambhar', 'rasam', curries and chutneys. These preparations are especially popular in the southern parts of India. Many parts of the tree are used in native medicines in Africa and Asia. The seeds are used in jam and jelly industry.

Precaution

Excessive use of tamarind is not advisable, as it may cause hyperacidity, cough and sexual weakness.

Turmeric

30

A Marvellous Medicinal Spice

Description

Turmeric *(Curcuma longa)* is a versatile natural plant. It combines the properties of a flavouring spice, a brilliant yellow dye, a natural beauty-aid and an effective household remedy for several diseases. It is a member of the ginger family Zingiberaceae. The Chinese name jianghuang literally means "yellow ginger."

Turmeric is a perennial plant, 60 to 90 cm in height, with an aerial short stem. It has raised or lifted branches and leaves which are held together at the base. The rhizomes are short and thick and they constitute the turmeric of commerce. It is largely consumed as a spice of daily use. The rhizhomes are dug up after the aerial stems have died, then washed, steamed and dried in the sun or oven.

Turmeric pieces are compact and heavy, having a yellow-brownish colour, and the outer surface is marked longitudinally with leaf-scars. The internal surface is dark-orange in colour and looks wet even though it is dry. Taste and smell of turmeric are aromatic.

Origin and distribution

Turmeric is a native of southern or South-Eastern Asia. It has been grown in India from ancient times and has been mentioned in early Sanskrit writings. It seems to have reached China before the seventh century A.D. Turmeric spread early throughout the East Indies and was carried eastwards across the pacific by Polynesians as far as Hawaii and Easter Island. It is mainly produced in India and other South-East Asian countries, including China. In India it is cultivated in almost all the states, particularly in Tamilnadu, West Bengal and Maharashtra.

Nutritive value/Composition

An analysis of turmeric shows it to consist of moisture 13.1 percent, protein 6.3 percent, fat 5.1 percent, minerals 3.5 percent, fibre 2.6 percent and carbohydrates 69.4 percent. Its mineral and vitamin contents are, calcium 150 mg. percent, phosphorous 282 mg. percent, iron 67.8 mg. percent, carotene 30 meg. percent, thiamine 0.03 mg. percent and niacin 2.3 mg. percent. Its calorific value is 349.

The main active ingredient of turmeric is curcumin which gives it its intense cadmium yellow colour. It is distributed through out the plant but, the dye is more concentrated in the rhizhomes. Dry rhizomes yield 5.8 percent essential oil, while the fresh ones yield 0.24 percent oil containing zingiberine. Ketone and alcohol are obtained on volatile distillation.

Medicinal virtues

Turmeric is truly one of the marvellous medicinal spices of the world. It has been used by Ayurvedic and Unani practitioners in India from time immemorial. It was prescribed by them as a drug to strengthen the stomach and

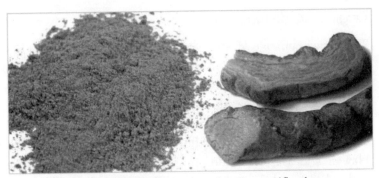

Turmeric is carminative, antiseptic, antiflatulant,
blood purifier and expectorant.

promote its action and also as a tonic and a blood purifier.
This spice is official in the Ayurvedic Pharmacopoeia of
India. It is also used extensively in traditional Chinese
medicine and is official in the Pharmacopoeia of the People's
Republic of China as well as in the Japanese Herbal Medicines
Codex.

Turmeric is aromatic, stimulant and a tonic. It corrects
disordered processes of nutrition and restores the normal
function of the system. It is useful in curing periodic
attacks. Turmeric is also carminative, antiseptic, antiflatulent, blood purifier and expectorant.

• Respiratory disorders

Turmeric is an effective household remedy for bronchial
asthma. The patient should be given a teaspoon of turmeric
powder with a glass of milk two or three times daily. It acts
best when taken on an empty stomach. Inhaling the fumes
of turmeric powder with tea leaves, blackgram and bengal
gram powder, reduces the spasms of asthma.

Turmeric is also valuable in bronchitis and tropical eosinophilia.
Half a teaspoon of turmeric powder and a pinch of coarsely
powdered pepper should be added to a glass of boiling milk.

It should be allowed to warm and used before going to bed as a medicine for treating bronchitis. For eosinophil, a teaspoon of turmeric powder, mixed with 30 gm of honey, should be taken thrice daily for three months.

• Intestinal disorders

Turmeric is a very useful intestinal antiseptic. The juice or dry powder of its rhizome, mixed in buttermilk or plain water, is beneficial in intestinal problems, especially chronic diarrhoea. It also helps prevent flatulence. The fresh juice from the rhizomes, a paste prepared from it or a decoction made from the plant has been found beneficial in the treatment of vomiting during pregnancy and affections of the liver. Turmeric has been found to inhibit bacterial growth and works as a powerful cleansing agent within the digestive system.

• Intestinal Worms

This spice is considered an effective remedy for expelling worms. About 20 drops of the juice of raw rhizomes, mixed with a pinch of salt, should be taken first thing in the morning daily in such cases. Another method to take turmeric for expelling worms is to mix half a teaspoon of turmeric powder and a pinch of salt in half a cup of lukewarm water on an empty stomach, once daily for 5 days.

• Anaemia

Turmeric, as a rich source of iron, is valuable in anaemia. A teaspoon of the juice from raw turmeric, mixed with honey, should be taken everyday in the treatment of this condition.

• Arthritis

This spice is a powerful anti-inflammatory food. Studies show that its primary compound curcumin is an anti-inflammatory agent on par with cortisone. It has been found to reduce inflammation in animals and symptoms of rheumatoid arthritis in humans. In an experiment, curcumin improved morning stiffness, walking time and joint swelling in 18 patients with rheumatoid arthritis. In fact, 1,200 mg of curcumin had the same anti-arthritis activity as 300 mg of the anti-inflammatory drug phenylbutazone.

• Measles

Turmeric is beneficial in the treatment of measles. Raw roots of the plant should be dried in the sun and ground to a fine powder. This powder, mixed with a few drops of honey and the juice of few bitter gourd leaves, should be given to the patient suffering from measles.

• Cold and cough

Turmeric, with its antiseptic properties, is an effective remedy for chronic cough and throat irritations. Half a teaspoon of fresh turmeric powder, mixed in 30 ml. of warm milk, is a useful prescription for treating these conditions. The powder should be put into a hot ladle. Milk should then be poured in it and boiled over slow fire. In case of a running cold, smoke from the burning turmeric should be inhaled. It will increase the discharge from the nose and bring quick relief.

For treating cough and allergy, a teaspoon of turmeric powder should be mixed in a cup of milk, and one pinch each of caraway seeds, pepper, cinnamon and dry ginger added to it. Then a cup of water should be added and the mixture boiled on a slow fire until the whole water is evaporated. This should be strained and taken daily before bed-time after adding some honey. This treatment should be continued for seven days.

Turmeric powder in combination with caraway seeds or

bishop's weed, is useful in colds in infants and children. A teaspoon of turmeric powder and a quarter teaspoon of caraway seeds or bishop's weed should be added to boiling water and the water should then be allowed to cool. About 30 ml. of this decoction, sweetened with honey, should be given thrice a day in treating this condition.

• Jaundice

The use of turmeric has been found beneficial in the treatment of jaundice. A pinch of turmeric powder should be taken along with a glass of hot water 2 or 3 times daily for a few days in this disease.

• Skin disorders

The fresh juice from the rhizomes is believed to have antiparasitic properties in many skin affections, especially ringworm and scabies. In a pilot study, conducted by the Medical and Cancer Research Treatment Centre of Nagercoil, India, turmeric paste was used for the treatment of scabies in 814 patients. The researchers concluded that turmeric paste is a very inexpensive, readily available, effective and acceptable mode of treatment for scabies without noticable toxicity or adverse reactions.

The fresh juice of raw turmeric can also be externally applied to the affected parts with beneficial results. Simultaneously, this juice, mixed with honey, should be taken orally. This juice as well as a paste prepared from the rhizomes and a decoction made from the plant are also considered useful as local application as well as internally in the treatment of leprosy.

• Mouth disorders

Turmeric is found beneficial in the treatment of oral disorders. A fine powder of charred turmeric used as a dentrifice with salt, is effective for relieving tooth ache. It prevents foul breath and dental caries.

• Boils

An application of turmeric powder to boils will speed up the healing process. In case of fresh boils, a few roots of the plant should be roasted and ash dissolved in a cup of water. The application of this solution will enable the boils to ripen and burst.

• Eye diseases

The use of turmeric is valuable in eye diseases, six gms of its powder should be boiled in 500 ml. of water till it is reduced to half. It should then be cooled. A few drops of this cold infusion can be used as eye drops in treating eye diseases.

• As beauty aid

A paste of turmeric applied on skin helps eliminate unwanted hair and improves complexion. A teaspoon of turmeric paste mixed with milk-cream, sandalwood paste and Bengal gram flour (besan) makes an excellent cosmetic. Applied once daily, it will keep the face fresh and soft.

A pinch of turmeric powder, mixed in the fresh leaf-juice of amaranth *(chaulai-ka-saag)* also serves as a valuable beauty-aid. Applied over the face, it bleaches the skin, prevents it from dryness and wrinkles, cures pimples and makes one look fresh. This juice, mixed with milk and lime juice, acts as an effective skin tonic to increase and retain its beauty. It should be delicately massaged over the face and neck for half an hour and washed with lukewarm water every night before going to bed.

A pinch of turmeric powder, mixed in a teaspoon of

coriander *(dhania)* juice, is also an effective remedy for pimples, blackheads and dry skin. The mixture should be applied to the face, after thoroughly washing it, every night before retiring.

Uses

Turmeric is an indispensable ingredient of the curry powder. It gives musky flavour and yellow color to curries. Curry powder usually contains 24 percent of turmeric powder. Turmeric powder is extensively used for its flavour and colour in butter, cheese, margarine, pickels, mustard and other food stuffs. It is also used to colour liquor, fruit drinks, cakes and jellies. Turmeric, both rhizomes and powder, is an auspicious article in all religious ceremonies in Hindu households. It is also an important dye in southern Asia. It can be used for dyeing cotton, silk and wool without a mordant, but the colour is fugitive. It is also used for colouring in pharmacy, confectionary and food industries.

Precaution

The *Botanical Safety Handbook* states that use of turmeric root should be avoided by people with bile duct obstruction or gallstones, it should not be administered to people who suffer from stomach ulcers or hyperacidity.

INDIAN NAMES OF SPICES AND CONDIMENTS

ENGLISH	HINDI	BENGALI	GUJARATI	KANNADA	MALAYALAM	MARATHI	TAMIL	TELUGU
Aniseed	Velaiti Saunf	Muhuri	Anisi	Sonpu	Shombu	Shep	Shombu	Sopuginja
Asafoetida	Hing	Hing	Hing	Hingu	Perungayam	Hing	Perungayam	Inguva
Basil	Tulsi	Tulsi	Tulsi	Vishpu tulsi	Trittavu	Tulshi	Thulasi	Thulasi
Bishop's Weeds	Ajwan	Joan	Ajamo	Oma	Ayamothakam	Onva	Omum	Vamu
Caraway Seeds	Shahi Jeera	Jira	Shahjiru	Shime Jeerige	Shima	Willayati	Shimal	Seema Sopyginjale
Cardamom	Elaichi	Elaychi	Elaychi	Yelakki	Elathari	Velchi	Elakkai	Elakkai
Celery	Ajwan-ka-patta	Randhumi	Ajma na pan Sag	—	Sellery	—	—	—
Chilli	Mirch	Lanka	Marcha	Menasina	Mulaku	Mirchi	Milagai	Mirapa Kayal
Cinnamon	Dalchini	Dalchini	Dalchini	Lavang eatti	—	Dalchini	Lavang Pattai	—
Clove	Laung	Lawang	Lavang	Lavanga	Grambu	Luvang	Kirambu	Lavangalu
Coriander	Dhania	Dhania	Dhania	Kothambari	Kothambalari	Dhane	Kothamalli Seeragam	Dhanivalu
Cumin Seed	Jira	Jira	Jiru	Jeerage	Jeerakam	Jira	Jeerkam	Jeelakarra
Curry Leaves	Curry Patta	Barsanga	Mitha Limbdo	Karibevu	Kariveppilai	Kadhi Limb	Kariveppilai	Karivepaku
Dill	Sowa	Sowa	Suva ni bhaji	Sabsige	Shatakuppa	Shepu	Satha kuppi	Sabsige
Fennel	Saunf, Sonp	Pan-Muhiri, Mauri	Variari	Badi—sopu	Perum-jeerakam	Badi—shep	Shombel	Sopu
Fenugreek	Methi	Methi	Methi	Menthya	Ventayan	Methi	Venthiya Keera	Menthulu

ENGLISH	HINDI	BENGALI	GUJARATI	KANNADA	MALAYALAM	MARATHI	TAMIL	TELUGU
Garlic	Adrak	Rashun	Lasan	Bellulli	Vellulli	Lasoon	Ullipoondu	Vellulli
Ginger	Adrak	Ada	Adu	Shunti	Inji	Ale	Inji	Allam
Liquorice	Mulethi	Jashti madu	Jethi mauch	Yashtima-dhukam	Iratimadhuram	Jyeshmadh	Atimadhuram	Yashti madhuka
Long Pepper	Pipal	Pipul	Lindi Pipper	—	Thippalli	Pimpali	Pipili	Pipallu
Marjoram	Mrarwa	Murru		Maruga	Maruvamu		Marru	
Mint	Pudina	Pudina	Fudina	Pudina	Pudina	Pudina	Pudina	Pudina
Mustard Seeds	Rai/Sarson	Sorse	Rai	Sasuve	Kadugu	Mohori	Kadugu	Avalu
Nutmeg	Jaiphal	Jaiphal	Jaiphal	Jajikai	Jathikka	Jaiphal	Jathikai	Jajikai
Onion	Piyaz	Pyaz	Kandoo/Dungari	Eerulli	Ulli	Kanda	Vengayam	Neerulli
Pepper	Kali Mirch	Kala Marich	Kalamari	Karemenasu	Kurumaluku	Mire	Milagu	Mirriyalu
Poppy Seeds	Khus Khus	Kaskash/Posto	Khuskhas	Khasksi	Khashakasha	Khus khus	Gasagasalu	Kasas Kasa
Saffron	Kesar	Jafran	Kesar	Kunkuma		Kesara	Kunkuma Poo	Kunkuma-puva
Tamarind	Imli	Tetul	Amli	Hunise Ambli	Puli	Chinch	Puli	Chintha Amlika
Turmeric	Haldi	Holud	Haldi	Anashina	Manjal	Halad	Manjal	Pasupu

Glossary of Medical and Botanical Terms

Abortifacient: An agent that promotes abortion.

Alopecia: A disease of the scalp resulting in complete or partial baldness.

Alterative: A drug which corrects disordered processes of nutrition and restore the normal function of an organ or of the system.

Amnesia: Forgetfulness

Analgesic: A drug which alleviates pain.

Anodyne: A drug that relieves pain.

Anthelmintic: A drug that kills intestinal worms.

Antipyretic: A drug which prevents or cures scurvy.

Antisapasmodic: A drug which counteracts spasmodic disorders.

Aperient: A mild purgative.

Aphrodisiac: A drug which promotes sexual desire.

Aromatic: Fragrant, spicy.

Astringent: A drug which arrests secretion or bleeding.

Axil: The angle formed by a leaf or branch with the stem of the plant.

Biennial: Living for two years under normal, outdoor conditions, usually producing seed in the second year.

Bulb: A subterranean leaf bud with fleshy scales or coats.

Camphor: A White, translucent, crystalline, swiftly-evaporating substance with an aromatic smell.

Carbuncle: An acute suppurative inflammation of the skin and tissues under the skin, rapidly spreading around the original point of infection.

Caries: Decay of teeth.

Carminative: A drug which relieves flatulence.

Cellulose: A shapeless white compound, insoluable in all ordinary solvents, forming the fundamental material of the structure of plants.

Chlorophyll: The green colouring matter of plants.

Colic: Pain due to spasmodic contraction of the abdomen.

Corm: The elongated fleshy base of a stem, ball-like but solid as in a saffron.

Cutin: A waxy substance which covers most of the aerial parts of vascular plants.

Cystitis: Inflammation of the bladder.

Decanted: Gradually poured from one container to another, without disturbing the sediment.

Decoction: A process of boiling down so as to extract some essence.

Demulcent: An agent that exercises a soothing effect on the skin and mucous membranes.

Diaphoretic: A drug that induces copious perspiration.

Diuretic: A drug which increases the secretion and discharge of urine.

Dymenorrhoea: Unusually painful and difficult menstruation.

Elliptical: Similar to oblong but with continuously rounding sides.

Emetic: A drug which induces vomiting.

Emollient: A durg which allays irritation of the skin and alleviates swelling and pain.

Emulsion: A fine dispersion of fatty liquid in another liquid, usually water.

Endocrine glands: Glands secreting directly into the blood stream—also known as ductless glands.

Endosperm: The stored food supply in the seeds.

Expectorant: A drug that promotes the removal of catarrhal matter and phlegm from the bronchial tubes.

Febrifuge: An agent used for reducing fever.

Flatulence: Excessive collection of gas in the stomach.

Floret: A small flower usually one of a dense cluster.

Genus: A classificatory group of animals or plants embracing one or more species.

Gonorrhoea: An infectious venereal disease marked by an inflammatory discharge from the genital organs.

Haemorrhage: Bleeding, especially profuse, from any part of the body.

Heartburn: A burning feeling in the regions of the chest and stomach, generally due to indigestion.

Hepatitis: Inflammation of the liver.

Infusion: A liquid obtained by steeping the herb, in liquid to extract the content.

Insulin: A hormone produced in the pancreas by the islets of Langherhans, regulating the amount of glucose in the blood and the lack of which causes diabetes.

Jaundice: A disease characterised by yellow discoloration of the skin and the tissues due to deposition in them of the pigment bilirubin.

Laxative: A drug which produces evacuated bowels.

Longevity: Length or duration of life.

Lumbago: A disease marked by severe pain in lower part of the back.

Mericarp: One of the two carpels that compose the fruit of a plant of the parsley or carrot family.

Micturition: Urination.

Mucilage: A sticky substance extracted from certain plants.

Narcotic: A drug which induces deep sleep.

Neuralgia: Pain felt along a nerve.

Nodule: A knot, lump, or node on the roots of plants.

Oblong: When nearly twice or thrice as long as broad and of uniform breadth.

Obtuse: With a blunt or rounded apex.

Oval: Broadly elliptical.

Ovate: Shaped like a lengthwise sector of a hen's egg. Somewhat oval with broader end downward.

Pericarp: The wall of the ovary or ovaries when developed or ripened into fruit, the mature ovary.

Petiole: The foot stalk or stem of the leaf.

Pharyngitis: Inflammation of the pharynx.

Pigment: Colouring matter, specially in the cell or tissue.

Poultice: A soft, medicated and usually heated mass applied to the body and kept in place with muslin, for relieving soreness and inflammation.

Rhizomes: An underground root like stem bearing both roots and shoots.

Rubefacient: A mild counter-irritant.

Sedative: A drug which reduces excitement, irritation and pain.

Sheath: A tubular envelop, as in the lower part of the leaf in grasses.

Species: A classifactory group of plants or animals subordinate to a genus and having members that differ only slightly among themselves.

Sperm: A mobile, celiated male reproductive cell.

Stigma: The part of the pistil which receives the pollen in pollination.

Stomachic: A drug that strengthens the stomach and promotes its action.

Style: The extended portion of a pistil connecting stigma and ovary.

Tannic Acid: A complex natural organic compound of a yellowish colour used as an astringent.

Tannin: An astringent chemical substance found in tea, coffee, and the barks of some trees.

Tuber: A short thickened underground stem having numerous buds or eyes.

Ulcer: An open sore on the skin.

Umbel: A flower cluster in which the flower stalk spring from the same point as in a wild carrot.

Umbelliferae: Having the mode of flowering called an umbel, a plant which bears umbel.

Uric acid: A crystalline acid forming a constituent of urine.

Volatile: Capable of rapid evaporation in air at ordinary temperature.

Whorl: A group of organs arranged about a stem, arising from the same node.

Bibliography

1. J.S. Pruthi, *Spices and Condiments,* National Book trust, India, New Delhi, 1987.

2. Jean Carper, *Food Your Miracle Medicine,* London, Simon & Schuster, 1995.

3. Bakhru H.K., *Healing Through Natural foods,* Jaico Publishing House, 2000.

4. Bakhru H.K., *Herbs That Heal, New Delhi,* Orient Paperbacks, 1998.

5. Oscar. Prof. Dr. Aman, *Medicinal Secrets of Your Food,* Mysore, Indo-American Hospital, 1985.

6. Kvj. Ganpati Singh Verma, *Miracles of Indian Herbs,* New Delhi, Rasayan Pharmacy, 1982.

7. Ceres Esplan, *Herbal Teas,* Northamptonshire, Thorsons Publishers Limited, 1986.

8. Dr. N. Ramaswami Pillai, *Herbal foods,* Nature-cure publishing House, Ganeshnagar, Pudukkottai, 1985.